Immunodeficiency
and
Disease

IMMUNOLOGY AND MEDICINE SERIES

IMMUNOLOGY
SERIES · SERIES · SERIES · SERIES **AND** SERIES · SERIES · SERIES · SERIES
MEDICINE

Immunodeficiency and Disease

Edited by
A. D. B. Webster
Consultant Physician
and Senior Scientist
Clinical Research Centre
Division of Immunological Medicine
Harrow, Middlesex
UK

Series Editor: Professor W. G. Reeves

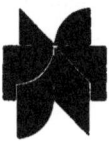

SPRINGER SCIENCE+BUSINESS MEDIA, LLC

British Library Cataloguing in Publication Data

Immunodeficiency and disease.
1. Man. Immune deficiency. Diseases
I. Webster, A. D. B.   II. Series
616.97'9

Library of Congress Cataloging-in-Publication Data

Immunodeficiency and disease / edited by A. D. B. Webster.
    p. cm. — (Immunology and medicine series)
    Includes bibliographies and index.
    ISBN 978-94-010-7066-9   ISBN 978-94-009-1275-5 (eBook)
    DOI 10.1007/978-94-009-1275-5
    1. Immunological deficiency syndromes.   I. Webster, A. D. B.
II. Series.
    [DNLM: 1. Immunologic Deficiency Syndromes.   WD 308 1335]
RC606.I48 1988
616.9'79—dc19
DNLM/DLC
for Library of Congress   88-12794
                                                                      CIP

Typeset by Witwell Ltd, Southport

Contents

Preface

The AIDS epidemic has popularized immune deficiency and has led to a rapid increase in the funding for research into the effect of viruses on immunity. There is now a real possibility of finding out whether some of the rare, so-called 'primary' immunodeficiency syndromes of children and adults, first described in the 1950s, may have a viral aetiology. Most of these syndromes have already been extensively reviewed more than once over the past 10 years, and their diagnosis and management is now included in most standard medical textbooks. In this volume, I have chosen to highlight what I consider to be the potentially exciting aspects of immunodeficiency in humans, hopefully providing clinicians and medical academics with some insight into the recent breakthroughs and disappointments.

There are three chapters discussing viral interactions with the immune system. Although much has been written about AIDS already, I make no apology for including an extensive review of both the clinical and laboratory aspects of this disease. AIDS is an important precedent, and it is likely that other less pathogenic retroviruses will eventually turn out to cause some of the rarer immunodeficiency disorders in children and adults. For instance, it has long been suspected that viruses may cause some of the non-familial types of severe combined immunodeficiency in infants; in fact HIV-1 infection now has to be considered in the differential diagnosis. By analogy with various animal diseases, there are some that believe that SLE, rheumatoid arthritis and other chronic inflammatory diseases might also be caused by retroviruses. Perhaps this is being over-optimistic, but it is important that clinicians are aware of this expanding field of research.

Of course, retroviruses are not the only 'devils in our midst' and the time is ripe for more research into the Epstein–Barr virus and cytomegalovirus. particularly since their molecular structure is now better understood. Immunologists, virologists and infectious disease clincians frequently see patients with protracted non-specific illness which they suspect is due to a chronic viral infection. Some of these patients show evidence of mild immunodeficiency. Using specific molecular probes, we should now be in a better position to clarify whether these patients have chronic herpes virus infections, either with well-known viruses or with some of the new recently isolated agents.

Dr Levin reviews the interferons, with particular emphasis on transient interferon deficiency during some viral infections. His work is not widely known by clinicians, and consequently there must be many patients still dying of fulminant virus infections without having had the benefit of interferon treatment. With new interferons being discovered and purified, much work needs to be done in the next decade to establish a therapeutic role for these antiviral and immunoregulatory substances.

There are two chapters on immunoglobulin (antibody) deficiencies. In their severe form these diseases are rare and probably only affect about 600 people in the United Kingdom. The aetiology of the acquired type has baffled clinical immunologists like myself for over 20 years. However, now that virologists and immunologists are working close together, evidence is emerging that this disease might have a retroviral cause. Furthermore, it has long been suspected that a small subgroup of these patients had EBV-induced hypo-gammaglobulinaemia, although definite proof has been lacking. New technologies will enable us to investigate this, as well as to test for the new lymphotropic herpes viruses which were discovered 'accidentally' in the blood of patients with AIDS and other disorders associated with immu-nosuppression.

What then is the aetiology and significance of selective IgA and IgG sub-class deficiencies, which probably occur in about 1 in 500 of the population? Hanson and Söderstrom's chapter shows how difficult it is to answer these questions. The association of these partial immunoglobulin deficiencies with disease remains largely anecdotal, and it is unlikely we shall understand their critical importance in host defence by investigating affected individuals in the western world. However, careful clinical studies in the third world, particularly in children, may demonstrate a role for IgA and IgG subclasses.

The chapter on severe combined and selective T cell deficiencies in infants and young children is devoted to two important genetically determined enzyme defects. Adenosine deaminase and purine phosphorylase are the only two enzymes so far known whose absence selectively compromises lymphocytes. Intuitively one suspects that the substrates or products of these enzymes are involved in immune regulation or the early development of the immune system. There are some interesting hypotheses, but a careful reading shows that a further, possibly serendipitous breakthrough is needed before we can understand why lymphocytes depend on these enzymes.

New autosomal recessive defects in the lymphocyte plasma membrane will probably be described in the next decade, particularly relating to activation signals for proliferation and differentiation. Although not reviewed here, absence of lymphocyte histocompatability antigens is a recent example of a membrane abnormality causing severe combined immunodeficiency.

Steady progress has been made over the past 10 years on our understanding of the complement pathway. Dr Walport highlights some of the recent excitements in this area, particularly the association of genetically determined defects of complement components and neutrophil complement receptors with connective tissue disorders or infections. Although the recognized complement receptor defects are very rare, it is likely that other defects will be discovered within the receptor complex; this will be of interest to both immunologists and those working on cell adhesion.

Dr Segal tells us about the hunt for the defect in chronic granulomatous disease. Although a rare inherited condition, this is an important experiment of nature because it will eventually tell us just how neutrophils kill bacteria. After a 15-year commitment to researching this disease, Dr Segal and his team are close to identifying the critical enzymes involved and cloning the relevant genes.

Some clinicians may find a few of the chapters too complicated and 'academic'. However, for those wishing to be experts in immunodeficiency there is no escape from having a thorough knowledge of the molecular abnormalities in these various syndromes. At least this will make those ward rounds that much more interesting.

A. D. B. Webster

Series Editor's Note

The modern clinician is expected to be the fount of all wisdom concerning conventional diagnosis and management relevant to his sphere of practice. In addition, he or she has the daunting task of comprehending and keeping pace with advances in basic science relevant to the pathogenesis of disease and ways in which these processes can be regulated or prevented. Immunology has grown from the era of antitoxins and serum sickness to a state where the study of many diverse cells and molecules has become integrated into a coherent scientific discipline with major implications for many common and crippling diseases prevalent throughout the world.

Many of today's practitioners received little or no specific training in immunology and what was taught is very likely to have been overtaken by subsequent developments. This series of titles on IMMUNOLOGY AND MEDICINE is designed to rectify this deficiency in the form of distilled packages of information which the busy clinician, pathologist or other health care professional will be able to open and enjoy.

Professor W. G. Reeves, FRCP, FRCPath
Department of Immunology
University Hospital, Queen's Medical Centre
Nottingham

List of Contributors

J. BJÖRKANDER
Department of Medicine I
University of Göteborg
Asthma and Allergy Research Center
Sahlgren's Hospital
S–41345 Göteborg
Sweden

D. A. CRAWFORD
Department of Virology
Royal Postgraduate Medical School
Hammersmith Hospital
Du Cane Road
London W12 ONN
UK

C. CUNNINGHAM-RUNDLES
Department of Medicine and Pediatrics
Mount Sinai Medical Center
One Gustave L. Levy Place
Box 1089
New York, NY 10029
USA

A. G. DALGLEISH
Division of Immunological Medicine
Clinical Research Center
Watford Road
Harrow, Middlesex HA1 3UJ

L. Å. HANSON
Department of Clinical Immunology
University of Göteborg
Guldhedsgatan 10
S–41346 Göteborg
Sweden

S. LEVIN
Department of Pediatrics and
Institute of Pediatric Research
Kaplan Hospital
Rehovat
76100
Israel

M. MALKOVSKY
Division of Immunological Medicine
Clinical Research Center
Watford Road
Harrow, Middlesex HA1 3UJ
UK

A. W. SEGAL
Department of Medicine
Rayne Institute
University College London
London WC1E 6JJ
UK

J. G. P. SISSONS
Department of Medicine
University of Cambridge
Level 5
Addenbrooke's Hospital
Hills Road
Cambridge CB2 2QQ
UK

R. SÖDERSTRÖM
Department of Medicine II
University of Göteborg
Asthma and Allergy Research Center
Sahlgren's Hospital
S–41345 Göteborg
Sweden

T. SÖDERSTRÖM
Department of Clinical Immunology
University of Göteborg
Guldhedsgatan 10
S–41346 Göteborg
Sweden

G. P. SPICKETT
Clinical Research Center
Division of Immunological Medicine
Watford Road
Harrow, Middlesex HA1 3UJ
UK

J. W. STOOP
Department of Pediatrics
University Hospital for Children and Youth
"Het Wilhelmina Kinderziekenhuis"
PO Box 18009
3501 CA Utrecht
The Netherlands

M. J. WALPORT
Rheumatology Unit
Department of Medicine
Royal Postgraduate Medical School
Du Cane Road
London W12 0NN
UK

A. D. B. WEBSTER
Clinical Research Center
Division of Immunological Medicine
Watford Road
Harrow, Middlesex HA1 3UJ
UK

B. J. M. ZEGERS
Department of Pediatric Immunology
University Hospital for Children and Youth
"Het Wilhelmina Kinderziekenhuis"
PO Box 18009
3501 CA Utrecht
The Netherlands

1
AIDS and the New Viruses

A. G. DALGLEISH AND M. MALKOVSKY

INTRODUCTION

In the beginning

The acquired immune deficiency syndrome (AIDS) was first recognized as a new disease entity in the spring of 1981, when clinicians in California and New York City notified the Centers for Disease Control (CDC) of the occurrence of *Pneumocystis carinii* pneumonia and Kaposi's sarcoma in previously healthy homosexual men. Similar cases with a variety of opportunistic infections, as well as non-Hodgkin's lymphomas, followed, and it rapidly became clear that the common feature in these patients was the presence of a cellular immune deficiency with no known underlying cause. The depiction of 'AIDS' as a new disease entity also allowed recognition that this was a new epidemic and not just a new diagnosis, as even with hindsight there is no evidence of possible cases occurring in or around the United States mainland until 1978 at the earliest[1-4].

Full descriptions of the syndrome, including typical opportunistic infections and neoplasms, were published in December 1981[5,6]; this showed that AIDS appeared to exclusively affect promiscuous homosexual men who reported very high numbers of sexual contacts (500–1000 per year) This 'risk group' did not remain exclusive for long as drug addicts and Haitians of both sexes developed AIDS. As the number of cases reported to the CDC began to rise exponentially it became obvious that AIDS was behaving as an infectious disease. Any doubts that were held were quickly dispelled with the transmission of the disease to haemophiliacs and recipients of blood and its products (some of whom were children)[7]. Although multiple infections from a single blood donor have been reported, haemophiliacs are of special note as some factor VIII and IX cryoprecipitate preparations are pooled from thousands of donors. The occurrence of AIDS outside the USA and Haiti was first recognized in homosexual communities in Western Europe, drug addicts, African immigrants and more recently Europeans returning from Africa. This led to the recognition of AIDS in Africa where it presented with

1

slightly different clinical features. It is now evident that AIDS is spreading epidemically throughout Africa and this will be discussed in more detail later[8].

A new form of persistent generalized lymphadenopathy (PGL; defined as the persistence of lymphadenopathy at two or more extrainguinal sites for 3 months or more in the absence of a defined cause) appeared at approximately the same time in the same at-risk populations. Similarly 'sick' at-risk persons who did not meet the diagnostic requirement for AIDS or PGL were also recognized. Their symptoms included severe wasting with weight loss and diarrhoea, intercurrent infections, night sweats, intermittent fever and general malaise; these patients were categorized as having AIDS-related complex (ARC). Since these conditions all occurred in the same at-risk populations and in some cases PGL or ARC symptoms preceded the development of AIDS, it became more likely that the causative agent may be associated with all the above categories of disease and that AIDS was the extreme end of the spectrum. This is now known to be the case[9,10].

The search for a cause

Having accepted that an infectious cause was the most likely, there was no shortage of possible contenders. Indeed early patients were infected with many known viruses, some of which are known to be immunosuppressive. Nevertheless, such candidates as cytomegalovirus (CMV), Epstein–Barr virus (EBV) and hepatitis B virus (HBV) were all well known to be associated with specific clinical disease patterns, none of which really resembled AIDS. It was far more likely that a new virus was the causative agent. But what type? To some virologists conversant with the many animal models of retrovirus disease and the discovery of the first human tumour retrovirus and causative agent of adult T-cell leukaemia (human T-lymphotropic virus – HTLV-I), a new human retrovirus seemed a likely contender[11]. Moreover, a similar virus was known to cause lymphosarcoma, aplastic anaemia, myelodysplastic anaemia and feline AIDS in cats[12]. This suggested that perhaps HTLV-I itself could cause AIDS, and indeed some AIDS patients were found to be HTLV-I seropositive.

First isolation of the causative agent

The history of 'who got there first' with regards to the first isolate has aroused controversy, although there is now general agreement on the sequence of events. The first publication of a new virus came from Luc Montagnier and co-workers at the Pasteur Institute who found a novel human retrovirus in a patient with PGL[13]. With only one isolate named LAV-I (*lymphadenopathy virus I*) and no significant serology, the aetiological association between virus and disease remained obscure until the successful multiple isolation and establishment of the virus in a permanent cell line by Robert Gallo and his colleagues[14]. This enabled enough virus to be produced to allow further characterization and a serological test. These isolates were named human T-cell lymphotropic viruses type III (HTLV-III), to distinguish them from other T-cell lymphotropic viruses, HTLV-I and HTLV-II[14]. Since these original reports, the virus has been variously called LAV, HTLV-III, a combination of both or AIDS-related virus (ARV)[15]. This situation has now been resolved by an international nomenclature committee declaring that the virus should be called the human immunodeficiency virus (HIV). Numerous isolates of HIV have now been obtained from all over the globe and a number of differences have been reported. Whereas most virus isolations have been made from peripheral blood lymphocytes, isolations have been reported from the bone marrow, lymph nodes, monocytes and macrophages, cell-free plasma, cerebrospinal fluid, semen, cervical fluid as well as from the cornea, tears, urine and the thymus[16].

CLINICAL FEATURES

Spectrum of disease

The clinical presentation of AIDS is diverse, encompassing a wide range of opportunistic infections and neoplasms (Table 1.1).

Table 1.1 Diseases moderately indicative of underlying immunodeficiency and seen in AIDS

Protozoal infection
   Pneumocystis carinii pneumonitis
   Toxoplasma gondii encephalitis or disseminated infection
   Chronic *Cryptosporidium* enteritis (> 1 month)

Fungal diseases
   Candida oral/oesophagitis/bronchitis
   Cryptococcal meningitis or disseminated infection
   Histoplasmosis (disseminated)
   Chronic enteric isosporiasis

Viruses
   Cytomegalovirus infection of an organ other than liver or lymph node
   Progressive multifocal leukoencephalopathy
   Herpes virus (chronic infection) – simplex or zoster
   Polyoma virus

Bacterial infection
   Mycobacterium avium complex or *M. kansasii* (and disseminated tuberculosis)
   Legionella sp.
   Nocardia sp.
   Salmonella sp.
   Shigella sp.
   Listeria monocytogenes

Helminthic infections
   Strongyloidiasis (disseminated beyond the gastrointestinal tract)

We now recognize that AIDS is the terminal manifestation of HIV-related disease. Following the initial infection, there may be a short glandular fever-like illness with seroconversion, after which the patient usually loses his

3

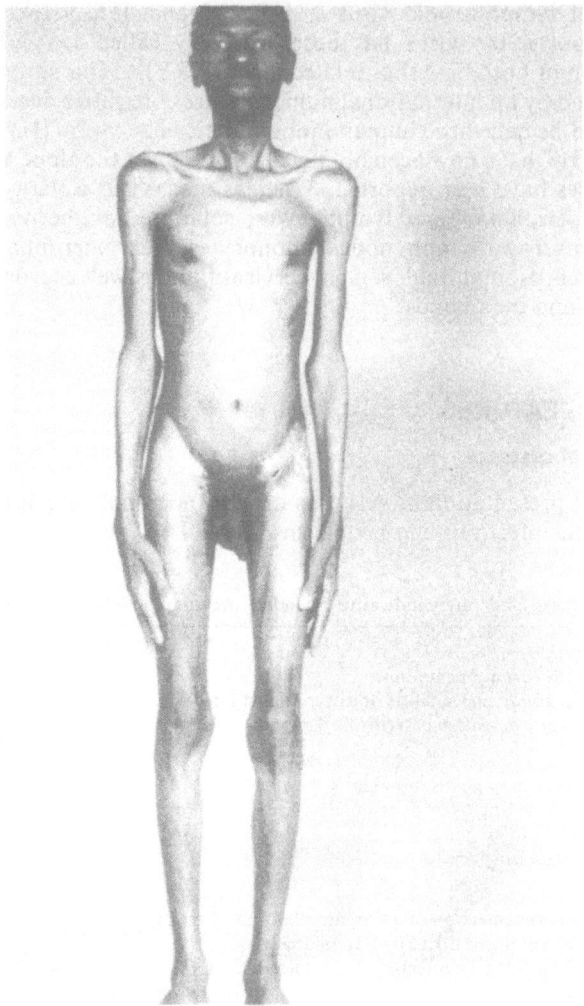

Figure 1.1 African man with 'Slim disease', showing marked weight loss and lymphadenopathy

symptoms[17]. Some patients then remain asymptomatic, whereas others develop ARC. The constellation of oral candidiasis, unexplained wasting and diarrhoea, referred to as pre-AIDS by some authors, resembles the clinical picture of HIV infection in Africa, where it is known locally as 'Slim disease' (Figure 1.1)[18].

Other conditions associated with HIV infection are severe skin disorders or dermatopathies. These include aggressive herpes simplex eruptions which ulcerate and haemorrhage. Herpes zoster, which may spread to involve more than one dermatome and cause intractable pain and blindness, is a further distressing complication. Hairy leukoplakia of the tongue is thought to

4

Table 1.2 Dermatological manifestations

Infections
   Herpes simplex
   Varicella zoster
   Pox virus:
      Molluscum contagiosum
   Papilloma virus:
      Verruca vulgaris
      Condyloma acuminatum

Fungi
   Candida albicans (thrush)
   Cryptococcus neoformans
   Histoplasma capsulatum
   Trichophyton rubrum

Protozoal
   Amoebiasis:
      Acanthamoeba castellani

Bacteria and mycobacteria
   Staphylococcus
   M. avium-intracellulare and *tuberculosis*

Malignancies
   Kaposi's sarcoma
   Hodgkin's and non-Hodgkin's lymphomas including Burkitt's lymphoma
   Squamous and basal cell carcinomas
   Cloacogenic carcinoma

Other
   Primary HIV infection
   Seborrhoeic dermatitis
   Oral 'hairy' leukoplakia
   Granuloma annulare-like eruption

Drug eruptions
   Sulphonamides
   Suramin

---

involve both EBV as well as papilloma virus. Perianal warts associated with papilloma virus infection and molluscum contagiosum involving the perineum are also being seen with increased frequency. Mycobacterium, candida and *Trichophytum rubrum* may cause florid skin disease, particularly in drug addicts (Table 1.2). Idiopathic thrombocytopenic purpura (ITP) can also be associated with HIV infection. It is often transient, probably autoimmune and responds poorly to prednisone in contrast to classical ITP[19].

Possibly the most disturbing symptoms are those of neurological disease which may present as florid dementia. Whereas this was first recognized in patients with AIDS, several neurological defects are now being reported in HIV seropositive patients with little or no other evidence of associated disease. Furthermore, a large number of HIV-infected patients can be shown to have some degree of neurological defect when appropriate tests are used[20] (Table 1.3).

Table 1.3 Neurological manifestations

Encephalitis
    viral
        HIV
        Cytomegalovirus
        Herpes simplex I, II and zoster
        Adenovirus
        Undetermined

    bacterial
        Treponema pallidum

    parasitic
        Toxoplasma gondii
        Taenia solium (cysticercosis)

Meningitis
    viral
        HIV or other

    bacterial
        M. tuberculosis
        M. avium-intracellulare
        E. coli
        Treponema pallidum
        Others

    fungal
        Cryptococcus neoformans
        Aspergillus fumigatus
        Histoplasma capsulatum
        Coccidioides immitis

Brain abcess
    bacterial
        Mycobacterium or other

    fungal
        Candida and others
    parasitic
        Toxoplasma gondii
        Taenia solium

Myelopathy
    viral
        HIV vacuolar myelopathy
        Cytomegalovirus
        Herpes simplex and zoster
        Epstein–Barr virus
        Others

    bacterial
        Syphilitic meningomyelitis

    compressive
        secondary to epidural abscess

Neuropathy
   viral
      HIV
      Cytomegalovirus
      Herpes simplex or zoster

Myositis of unknown origin

Progressive multifocal leukoencephalopathy (secondary to papovavirus)

Neoplastic
   Brain lymphoma
   Metastatic disease (including
     carcinomatous meningitis and
     compressive myelopathy)
   Lymphomas
   Kaposi's sarcoma
   Plasmacytoma sarcoma
   Sarcoma

Vascular complications
   Haemorrhage secondary to immune
     thrombocytopenia
   Embolic stroke secondary to marantic
     endocarditis
   Parainfectious cerebral arteritis
   Vascular compromise secondary to *Aspergillus fumigatus infection*

Metabolic disorders
   drug effects
   electrolyte
   vitamin deficiency

AIDS

The major opportunistic infections comprise *Pneumocystis carinii* pneumonia (PCP), disseminated cytomegalo and Herpes simplex virus infections, mucosal candidiasis, cerebral toxoplasmosis, disseminated mycobacterial infections (*M. avium-intracellulare, M. tuberculosis*), cryptococcosis, salmonellosis and cryptosporidiosis (see Table 1.1). The exact nature of the opportunistic disease tends to reflect to some degree the organisms prevalent in the environment, especially those which are latent in or carried by the host. This accounts for regional and geographical variations in the opportunistic infections seen, such as a high prevalence of salmonella infection in the UK and Europe and the different pattern of atypical mycobacteria in the UK (*M. xenopii* and *M. kansasii*). *M. tuberculosis* is one of the commonest pathogens in HIV patients in some parts of Africa. Histoplasmosis and coccidiomycosis are seen in patients who come from those areas in North America where these infections are prevalent.

In some respects, the pattern of infections and malignancies are reminiscent of that seen in patients with congenital or acquired cellular immune deficiency, such as children with severe combined immune deficiency or recipients of high dose corticosteroids after renal transplantation or patients with systemic lupus erythematosus (SLE). However, the presentation and response to treatment of these infections is often different in AIDS. For example, pneumocystis infections proceed insidiously over several weeks rather than the rapidly over a few days as in other immunocompromised patients. Although the clinical and radiological signs may be mild, the organism is usually present in large numbers in bronchial lavage fluid. Furthermore, the response to treatment (high dose Septrin or Pentamidine) may be transient with recrudescence upon cessation of therapy, and has a 30% failure rate. Further complications may arise due to a high rate of sensitization to co-trimoxazole. However, prophylactic treatment with co-trimoxazole, if tolerated, or sulphadoxine/pyrimethamine (Fansidar), would appear to reduce recurrence.

The clinical picture of atypical mycobacterial disease resembles the picture seen in lepromatous leprosy, with negligible host defence and a large number of organisms. It is often resistant to common antituberculous drugs. Cytomegalovirus (CMV) infections cause a more diffuse and disseminated disease than that seen in non-AIDS patients with the additional complications of malabsorption and colitis, adrenal insufficiency and progressive chorioretinitis which may impair vision. Toxoplasmosis, like CMV, is difficult to diagnose serologically because of high non-specifically raised antibody titres. This may involve the brain where it may be difficult to

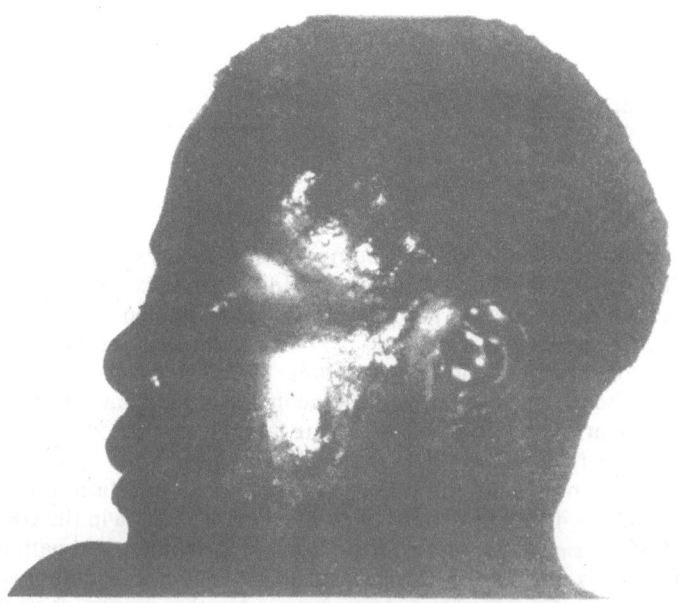

Figure 1.2 An aggressive type of Kaposi's sarcoma in an African man with AIDS

differentiate from a cerebral lymphoma, which also has a high incidence in AIDS.

Cryptococcus neoformans may cause a diffuse pneumonitis, meningitis or encephalitis. Often it is widely disseminated and may present with granulocytopenia, lymphopenia and thrombocytopenia, ulcerating gastrointestinal lesions and fever. Oral candidiasis is common and oesophageal involvement may present with dysphagia and retrosternal burning. It may require systemic Amphotericin B to resolve lesions.

Intractable diarrhoea is also a major problem and may be due to many infectious causes such as salmonella, *Giardia lamblia*, shigella and cryptosporidium, as well as malignant infiltration with Kaposi's sarcoma (KS) or lymphoma. An important feature, however, is that extensive investigation may fail to document a causative organism in many patients.

Cerebral manifestations of toxoplasmosis and cerebral lymphomas have already been mentioned, but it should be noted that many other cerebral complications, such as CMV involvement and progressive multifocal leukoencephalopathy, have been reported. Nevertheless, the increasing recognition of direct HIV infection of brain tissue itself suggests that the virus can cause dementia[20].

AIDS and malignancy

Kaposi's sarcoma (KS) occurs in up to 30% of patients with AIDS, although there is a considerable difference between different at-risk groups. Most of the reported cases are homosexual patients, whereas it is very rare in haemophiliacs and drug addicts. The clinical presentation encompasses a broad spectrum from indolent lesions to widespread involvement of the skin (Figure 1.2). However, internal organs, especiall those of the gastrointestinal tract, may be involved in HIV-infected patients, resulting in constriction or obstruction of the oesophagus and/or trachea. The mucosa of the oral cavity is often affected and the lesions appear as dark blue purple colorations. The detailed classification of KS is more extensively reviewed by Dalgleish and Weiss[9]. When it is not associated with AIDS, KS usually occurs in elderly males of Mediterranean or Jewish origin, in whom it is typically confined to the lower limbs and does not cause any significant morbidity or mortality. This benign form also occurs in Africa as well as a rapidly progressive type. It has been suggested that KS in AIDS patients is an opportunistic neoplasm associated with a latent viral infection. Interestingly, the incidence of KS in other immunocompromised hosts is very low which suggests that other factors are involved in HIV-infected individuals.

An earlier suggestion that CMV may be the causative agent is not supported by molecular hybridization studies. Furthermore, there is no evidence of the HIV genome in the lesions.

The pathogenesis of KS is still poorly understood and even its classification as a malignancy is much debated. Proliferating endothelial cells appear to be the primarily involved cells in the KS lesion. Endothelial cells are not known to be infectable with HIV, although they are subject to control by subsets of helper (CD4+) T lymphocytes which are compromised in HIV infection.

The clinical management of KS in patients with AIDS is notoriously difficult, mainly because the disease has such a diverse course and it is difficult to be sure whether or not therapy has been effective. The indolent form is responsive to both radiotherapy and simple chemotherapy, whereas the aggressive variety in AIDS and African patients is relatively resistant. Although aggressive multidrug regimens have a better response rate than single agents, the added toxicity of therapy appears to be detrimental. Indeed, Vinblastine or VP16 alone is now the preferred treatment, with the object of control rather than cure.

Lymphomas

The association of B-cell non-Hodgkin's lymphoma (NHL) with HIV infection is now well established. Hodgkin's disease may also be more common, which has prompted speculation that this too may have a viral cause[21]. As is the case with KS, the highest incidence of NHL is in homosexual men. The histological features are of intermediate differentiated and immunoblastic malignant lymphoma of B-cell type. A progression from polyclonal B-cell hyperplasia to monoclonal B-cell neoplasia has been documented by several authors.

Activation of EBV is one possible explanation. This herpes virus can usually be isolated from patients with AIDS, as it can from many healthy subjects, but the tumours show no evidence of EBV involvement at the molecular level. The current theory of lymphomagenesis suggests a sequence of genetic changes involving activation or alteration of oncogenes (e.g. myc). Amplified gene activity, presumably affecting cellular growth factors, then provokes neoplastic change[22]. Some authors have implicated a critical role for suppressor T cells in this process on the basis of the observations that lymphomas may regress when drug immunosuppression is withdrawn (in transplant patients). Recently it has been noted that some AIDS patients with NHL are also infected with HTLV-I, which has a well documented association with lymphomas in humans. HTLV-I immortalizes T cells and a second 'genetic' event could provoke monoclonal neoplasia.

The proclivity of NHL to affect the brain has already been mentioned, and this may be the only involved site at presentation. Response to classical NHL treatment in HIV-infected patients is extremely poor and the disease is usually very aggressive.

Both Hodgkin's disease and other malignancies are being seen with increased frequency in 'AIDS at-risk' populations which are not necessarily infected with HIV. These include squamous carcinoma of the oral cavity and cloacogenic carcinoma of the rectum which may be caused by papilloma viruses similar to those associated with cancer of the cervix.

THE VIRUS

Retroviruses are RNA-containing viruses that replicate through a DNA intermediate. Both RNA and DNA contain all the genetic information of the retrovirus. However, the ends of retroviral RNA differ from those of its DNA counterpart. The RNA has a small terminal repeat, which is important for the synthesis of viral DNA, whereas the DNA has a long terminal repeat (LTR).

Retroviruses encode an enzyme, reverse transcriptase, which allows them to use the replicative machinery of the host cell. The HIV family of viruses displays the general properties of retroviruses:

(1) 5'LTR-gag-pol-env-3'LTR genomic organization;

(2) Presence of a unique non-structural protein necessary for replication – the enzyme reverse transcriptase (RNA-dependent DNA synthetase), which is similar to the reverse transcriptases of other retroviruses;

(3) High molecular weight RNA;

(4) Glycoprotein envelope;

(5) Budding at the cell surface.

The retroviruses are divided into three subgroups – oncoviruses, lentiviruses and spumaviruses. The oncoviruses have oncogenic potential, while the spumaviruses cause inapparent disease in animals and vacuolization of cultured cells. The lentiviruses, including visna virus, equine infectious anaemia virus (EIAV) and caprine arthritis and encephalitis virus (CAEV), display many structural and biological parallels with HIV to such an extent that the latter is now classified as a lentivirus.

The common features of lentiviruses are as follows:

(1) Persistent infection;

(2) Proviral complementary DNA is not only integrated in the host's genome but is also found in the cytosol as circular or linear double-stranded DNA;

(3) Cytopathic effect *in vitro*.

Mature HIV virions are 110–130 nm in diameter and have a small electron dense core which is, depending on the plane of section, round or bar-shaped. They are not seen on electron microscopy until budding has commenced at the cell surface.

HIV virions contain several antigenic proteins. The precursor protein p55 and its cleavage products, p12, p16 and p24 are associated with the core. The p24 is the major antigenic protein of HIV. The major envelope protein, gp110 (also referred to as gp120), is glycosylated. Antibodies against this glycoprotein also recognize its cleavage products, gp70, gp41 and gp34. The sera of most persons infected with HIV contain antibodies against the core and envelope proteins, whereas antibodies against other antigenic proteins of HIV have been detected less frequently.

In order to infect, the virus must first enter a permissive cell, usually by means of a specific receptor. After adhesion to this receptor the virus receptor/complex undergoes invagination into the cytoplasma of the cell,

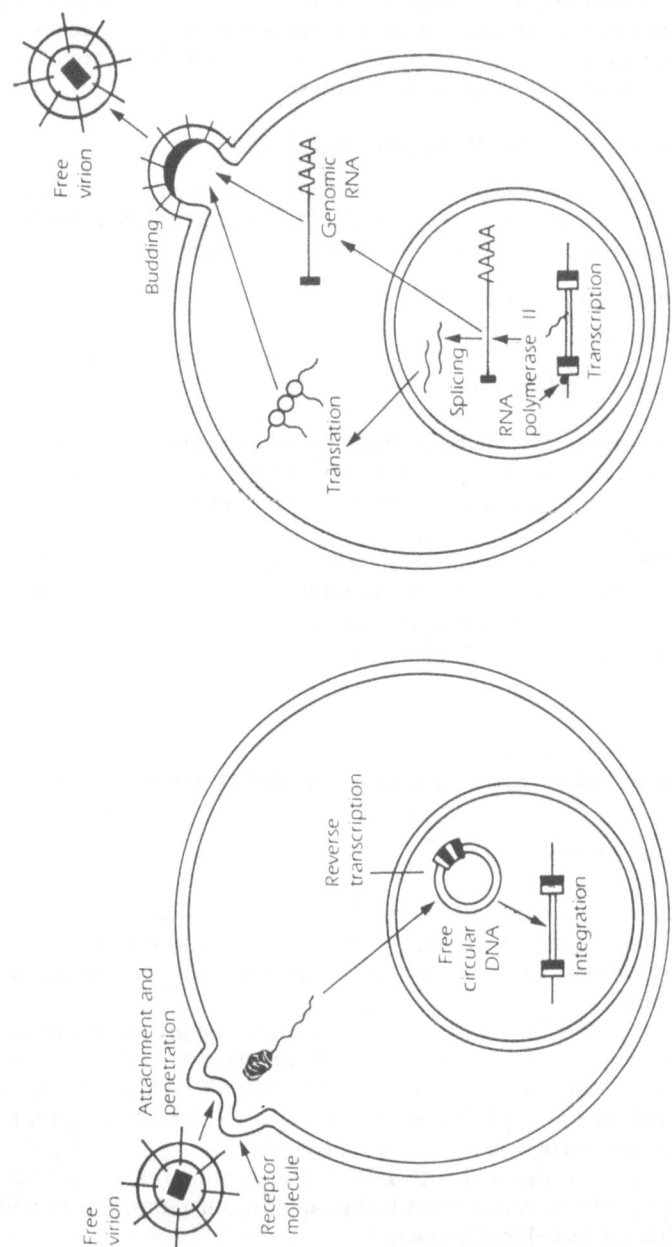

Figure 1.3 Diagram representing the attachment, integration and replication of HIV

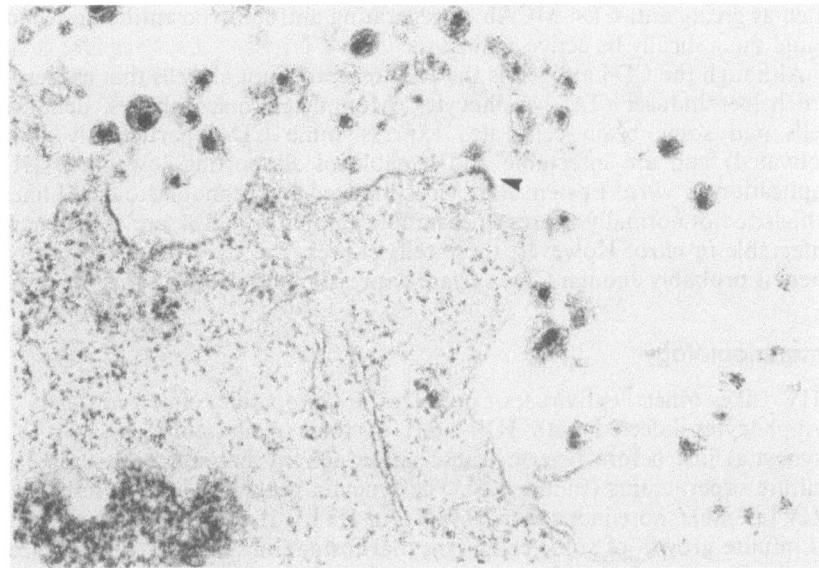

Figure 1.4 HIV particles budding from the surface (arrow) of a CD4⁺ lymphoblastoid cell line (× 32000)

where it is packaged in an endosome. This then fuses with a lysosome in which the virus becomes uncoated; infectious RNA is released and starts a new life cycle (Figures 1.3 and 1.4).

The receptor

Early studies showed that the number of circulating T4 (helper/inducer) lymphocytes was markedly depressed in patients with AIDS or at-risk for AIDS[8]. The CD4 (or T4) antigen was shown to be the receptor for HIV-I by testing 160 monoclonal antibodies (MCAb) to leukocyte antigens in infectivity assays. All the anti-CD4 MCAb blocked infection. Down regulation of the CD4 antigen also occurs following infection with HIV. No other component of the receptor has yet been identified even though it is very unusual for a virus to be so restricted to one receptor. Transfection studies, where the cloned CD4 gene is inserted into CD4-negative human cells (e.g. epithelial cells) have clearly shown that they are rendered infectable with HIV after expressing the CD4 antigen. Some healthy people have subtle variations in the CD4 antigen, and antibodies to some of these different epitopes do not block HIV infection of CD4+ cells *in vitro*. However, a study of CD4 epitope polymorphism in AIDS at-risk people of African and Caucasian origin found no correlation between the development of AIDS in these two groups. Moreover, the fact that different epitopes of CD4 are involved in HIV infection has enabled a rough epitope map to be made using competition blocking assays. This may be useful in designing future therapeutic strategies such as giving anti-CD4 MCAb or generating anti-idiotype antibodies which could theoretically be active against the virus[23,24].

Although the CD4 antigen is the HIV receptor, not all cells that express it are helper/inducer (T4) lymphocytes. Monocytes, macrophages, dendritic cells and some brain cells also express some CD4 (particularly when activated) and are infectable and capable of supporting low grade HIV replication *in vitro*. Epstein-Barr virus-induced B lymphoblastoid cell lines, which do not normally express measurable amounts of CD4, are occasionally infectable *in vitro*. However, these cells express the CD4 RNA message so there is probably enough CD4 surface expression to facilitate virus binding.

Immunobiology

HIV, like other lentiviruses, produces a cytopathic effect *in vitro*. T lymphocytes infected with HIV start to form giant multinucleated cells (syncytia) just before reverse transcriptase activity becomes measurable in culture supernatants (Figure 1.5). The syncytia generated in the presence of HIV resemble those induced by HTLV-I or HTLV-II, but instead of initiation of infinite growth of some cells, syncytial formation is accompanied by cell death. This correlates with expression of viral envelope antigen. But what causes the cell death? Activation of a cytotoxic protein, acceleration of cell senescence and interactions between viral proteins and the CD4 molecule have all been proposed. Another possibility is that cell death is due to the accumulation of large amounts of intracellular viral DNA and RNA. The

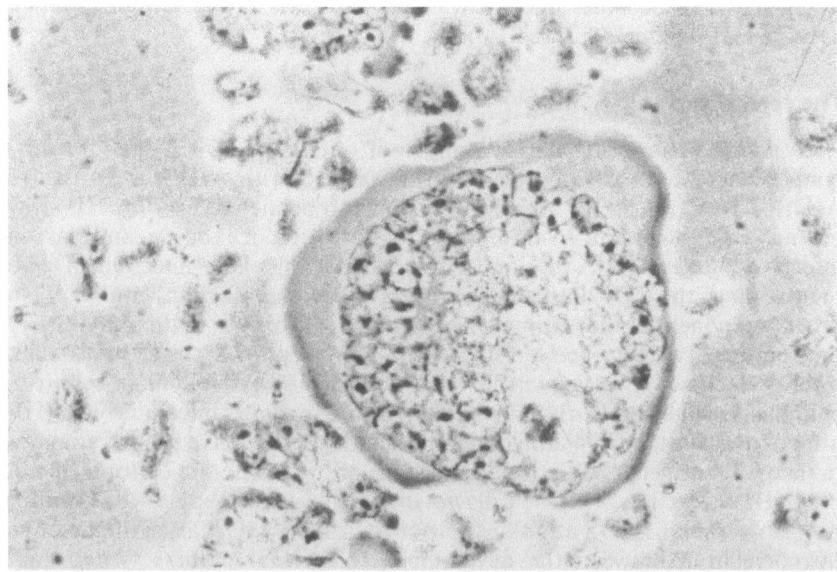

Figure 1.5 Syncytial formation in a CD4+ lymphoblastoid cell line. The large cell is made up of many fused lymphoblastoid cells, their nuclei remaining visible

mystery is even more puzzling in the light of a finding by Hoxie *et al.* (1985)[25] that some T cells cultured in medium supplemented with interleukin 2 (IL-2) remain productively infected with HIV without showing any cytopathic effect.

HIV infection eventually leads to a marked decrease in the numbers of helper/inducer T4-positive lymphocytes, and often elevated numbers of suppressor/cytotoxic T8-positive lymphocytes. A possible explanation for this phenomenon is that the T4 population is destroyed by HIV, and the T8 cells are stimulated by an active Epstein-Barr or cytomegalovirus infection, which occurs in more than 90% of AIDS patients. In this context it may be relevant that T cells from these patients often spontaneously proliferate when cultured *in vitro*. Recent evidence suggests that viral expression by proliferating T cells is controlled by T8+ cells[26]. Clinically reduced numbers of T4 cells are accompanied by an increased host susceptibility to both bacterial and viral infections (particularly opportunistic infections such as *Pneumocystis carinii* pneumonia or cytomegalovirus retinitis), and neoplasms such as Kaposi's sarcoma and lymphomas. Can these symptoms be explained by the T-helper cell involvement alone?

HIV-infected persons tend to show decreased delayed-type hypersensitivity responses *in vivo*. For instance, using seven skin-test antigens, the number of positive responses was only about 25% of that in a healthy control group[3]. It is not clear whether this is due to low numbers of T4 cells or involvement of another cell (e.g. macrophage) which are important in delayed hypersensitivity reactions.

T cells isolated from peripheral blood of HIV-infected persons usually show a decrease in (1) proliferative responses to mitogens and antigens, (2) cytotoxic functions, (3) helper activities for B lymphocytes, (4) the expression of the receptor for IL-2, and (5) the production of IL-2. These defects could be due to non-specific suppressive molecules released from HIV-infected T cells[27], in a similar way to factors produced after immunization, which probably limit the entry of new cells into an immune response[28]. Such a mechanism could be inappropriately activated in AIDS patients.

An interesting feature of the humoral response in AIDS is the apparent polyclonal B-cell activation. This is manifested by (1) elevated levels of serum immunoglobulins and circulating immune complexes, (2) increased numbers of spontaneous plaque-forming cells in the peripheral blood, (3) an augmented spontaneous proliferation of B lymphocytes and hyperresponsiveness to B-cell growth factors *in vitro*, (4) meagre or absent antigen-specific antibody responses following immunization, and (5) failure to respond to some activation signals *in vitro*. A direct polyclonal activation of human B lymphocytes by HIV in the absence of the normal regulatory T-cell environment could partly explain these abnormalities[29].

The number of monocytes in the peripheral blood of AIDS patients is usually normal, although the number of monocytes bearing the CD4 molecule decreases in line with the T4 helper cells. Their monocytes are also normal with respect to phagocytosis, intracellular killing of micro-organisms and enhancement of H_2O_2 release and cytotoxicity in response to γ-interferon. However, their chemotactic activity is markedly decreased, especially in the later stages of disease. Furthermore, patients with AIDS display a substantially decreased rate of removal of autologous erythrocytes coated with anti-Rh antibodies, implying a defect in Fc receptor-mediated clearance; this may be due to the blockage of Fc receptors by circulating immue complexes. Langerhans' cells from AIDS patients are deficient in the expression of HLA class II molecules, but their immunological competence has not been studied.

In contrast to some primary T-cell immunodeficiencies in young children, increased α_1-thymosin levels have been detected in patients with AIDS and healthy homosexual men. Also β_2-microglobulin is increased. β_2-microglobulin is the light chain of HLA class I molecules, which are present on the surface of practically all cells in the body. The increase in serum levels could reflect a higher rate of lymphocyte cell-membrane turnover and signal the development of clinical deterioration in HIV infection.

Virus neutralization

Whereas most viruses, including HTLV-1 and HTLV-2, induce strong neutralizing antibodies, HIV induces only a very weak neutralizing response even though the response to a variety of antigens in the viral envelope is vigorous. Other viruses which fail to induce neutralizing antibodies have a low virion number and tend to 'hide' in macrophages. Another possibility is that the neutralizing epitope is hidden by other antigens. This, together with differences in the envelope antigen between different HIV isolates will make it difficult to produce a useful vaccine. However, all isolates so far tested bind to the T4 molecule which shows that there is a conserved structure in the envelope and that vaccines should be directed towards antibodies to this epitope.

Molecular biology

The HIV particle contains two identical molecules of genomic RNA. The complete HIV genome has been cloned as DNA and sequenced. HIV does not contain any DNA which is homologous to the DNA found in the human genome and integration of HIV proviruses does not occur at specific sites in the host cell genome. The lengths of proviral DNAs sequenced independently by four research groups are in the range of 9193–9749 base pairs (bp)[30].

The sequences that encode viral proteins (Figure 1.6) are flanked by LTRs (long terminal repeats). The LTRs contain signals that participate in the integration of viral DNA into the host genome and in the regulation of transcription of viral genes (viral RNA synthesis).

The genome of HIV, like that of other retroviruses, contains three open reading frames, *gag*, *env* and *pol*, which encode the capsid (core) proteins, the envelope proteins and Mg^{2+}-dependent reverse transcriptase, respectively. In addition, the HIV genome contains at least five other open reading frames, *sor*, R, *tat-III*, *art* and *3′orf*, which are not common to most retroviruses.

The *gag* open reading frame contains the *gag* gene (~512 condons) which encodes the internal structural proteins of the virion. The precursor

16

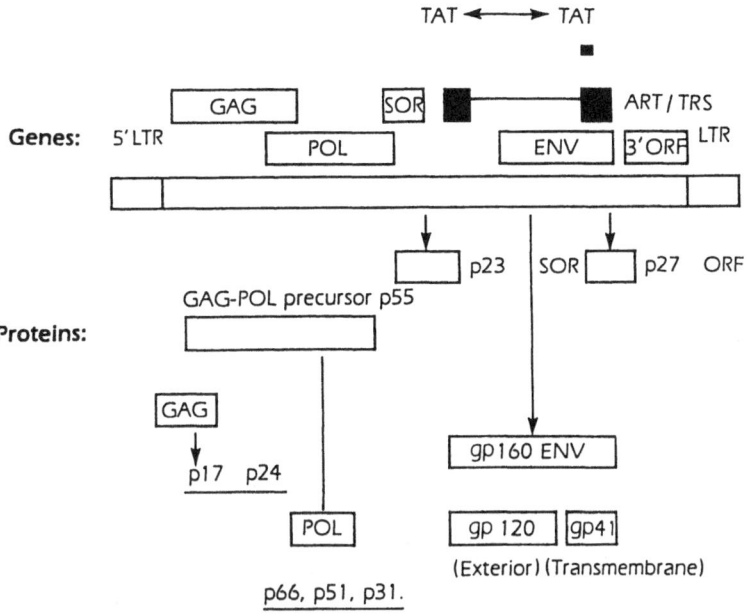

Figure 1.6 The genes and proteins of HIV

polypeptide, p55, is synthetized and cleaved to yield mature *gag* proteins, p24 and p17, which are well conserved amongst HIV isolates; these are the antigens most likely to be detected by available commercial assays.

The *pol* open reading frame (~1003 codons) overlaps the *gag* open reading frame by 80 amino acids. It has numerous regions where the predicted amino acid sequence shows considerable homology to *pol* gene products of HTLV-I, Rous sarcoma and murine leukaemia viruses.

The *env* open reading frame can code a protein 863 amino acids long. The *env* gene encodes the major glycoprotein found in the envelope of the virus and in the cytoplasmic membrane of infected cells. The size of the predicted products is in accordance with the detection of a 120 kDa envelope glycoprotein, and virion-associated gp41 which is the transmembrane protein.

The *sor* (short open reading frame) gene encodes a 23 kDa protein. The *3'orf* (open reading frame) extends into the 3-LTR, consists of three exons and codes for a 27 kDa protein. The function of the R, *sor* and *3'orf* genes and their products is a subject of speculation.

The *tat-III* (trans-activating transcriptional regulation) gene also consists of three exons, the first of which does not code for protein structure. Its transcription into a functional messenger RNA (mRNA) involves double splicing which brings together sequences from the 5' part (287 bp), middle (268 bp) and 3' part (1258 bp) of the HIV genome. The second and third exon code for the *tat-III* protein (86 amino acids). The second exon, which codes for 72 amino acids and represents the major functional domain of the trans-activator gene, is located between the *sor* and *env* genes, in a region orginally thought to be non-coding. The remaining 14 amino acids are coded by a small exon within the *env* gene. The *tat-III* gene product stimulates LTR-directed gene expression through the interaction with specific sequences (TAR) in the leader of viral messages. Mutations in the 5' portion of the first coding exon result in inefficient synthesis of structural proteins and hinder virus replication. Similar trans-acting factors in HTLV-I, HTLV-II and bovine leukaemia virus (BLV) are products of a viral gene termed *tat* or *x-lor*.

The observation that diminished expression of *gag* and *env* proteins associated with mutations near the two coding exons of the *tat-III* gene cannot be corrected by the *tat-III* gene product alone suggests the existence of another trans-activator gene. It is postulated that the coding exons of this gene use alternative reading frames of both coding exons of the *tat-III* gene. The splicing events needed to generate this alternative reading frame product are essentially the same as those required for the *tat-III* gene expression. The product of the alternative reading frame is 116 amino acids long and contains a number of basic hydrophilic residues similar to those found in the *tat-III* gene product as well as in other nucleic acid-binding proteins. The gene was named *art* (anti-repression trans-activator). The proposed function of its product is to neutralize the effects of *cis*-acting negative-regulatory sequences present on viral mRNA coding for the HIV structural proteins[31].

Although the genomic diversity of HIV is well documented[30], proviral DNAs from different HIV isolates hybridize with each other even under high stringency conditions. The most divergent part of the HIV genome is the part of the *env* gene coding for the exterior glycoprotein. HIV isolates differing from each other in 20% of amino acids encoded by the *env* gene are common. The genetic variability of HIV could reflect a selective advantage of mutations, for instance on the basis of a 'sneaking through the immue response' mechanism similar to that of EIAV in horses.

THE EPIDEMIOLOGY OF AIDS

The first reports of AIDS were published in the Morbidity and Mortality Weekly Report in June and July 1981, and from this time surveillance was initiated throughout the United States. The first 1000 patients were reported in February 1983 (over 5 years after the onset of disease in the first recognized cases), the 2nd 1000 cases by July 1983 and the 3rd by December 1983; since then the numbers have continued to rise exponentially and by the end of 1986 there were nearly 30 000 cases in the USA. Similar patterns have been seen in other countries, in that a few cases are reported in the first few years followed by a rapid doubling (between 5 and 12 months) in the subsequent years.

Whereas the first cases were recognized in promiscous homosexuals, haemophiliacs, Haitians and intravenous drug abusers, the group at risk is now much larger and includes heterosexually active adults and children of seropositive mothers.

The Haitian connection was difficult to explain initially although it is now clear that Haiti is a popular vacation resort for New York homosexuals who consorted with local bisexual males. Documented transmission of AIDS in heterosexual couples in the US began to apper in 1983 and a year later in Africa. Transmission has been documented from male to female and female to male, implicating prostitutes as a potential reservoir for the spread of the disease. However, relatively few females have transmitted the disease to males in the USA. This may be due to the relatively low numbers of females at present infected or may represent a less efficient route of transmission (cf. gonococcal infections). However, a recent survey shows that 40% of HIV seropositive people in Manhattan are female, so the rate of female-to-male spread is likely to rise.

AIDS and Africa

AIDS was recognized in African patients being treated in Brussels and Paris in 1983, many of these patients being from Rwanda and Zaire (Figure 1.7). Surveys subsequently showed that there was an epidemic of AIDS in the heterosexual population, particularly in prostitues. The clinical features of AIDS in Africa are often different from the West. This is probably due to the different spectrum of opportunistic organisms in the environment.

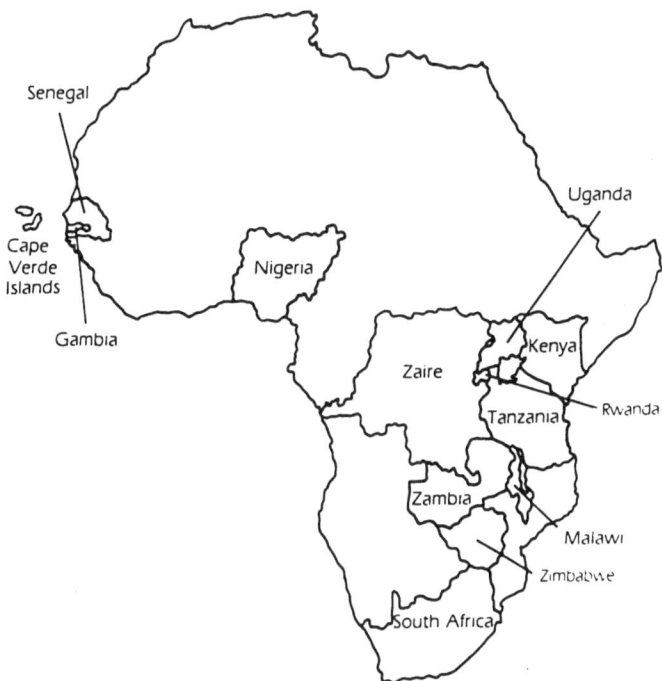

Figure 1.7   African states where human retroviruses have frequently been detected

19

Tuberculosis is becoming a major problem in patients with HIV infection, and a syndrome of wasting fever and diarrhoea (Slim disease) is a common presentation in some parts of Africa. Kaposi's sarcoma (KS) occurs in up to 40% of African patients with HIV infection. There is an endemic variety of KS, not related to AIDS, which is a slow indolent disease in elderly males affecting the limbs and rarely causing death. However, HIV infection is associated with a very aggressive form of KS, sometimes causing death within 12 months[32,33].

How long has AIDS been in Africa?

Clinicians who have worked in Africa since the 1960s are sure that AIDS is a new epidemic. However, a few African patients with a clinical diagnosis compatible with AIDS were treated in European clinics in the early 1970s, and in a retrospective survey of 700 sera collected in 1959 from Africans, one was definitely positive. Nevertheless, the rapid spread of the disease has been relatively recent, occurring initially in Kigali, Rwanda and Kinshasa in Zaire in 1980, and then in Zambia and Uganda in 1982, from where it has spread to other areas in Central Africa. A similar virus (STLV-III) to HIV has been found in asymptomatic African Green monkeys, both in those living in the US for more than 20 years and those caught in the wild in Africa. The recent isolation and identification of an HIV variant in healthy Senegalese prostitutes by Essex and co-workers appears to be closer to STLV-III than HIV on immunoblotting. This new human virus has been called HTLV-4. A French group have isolated a similar virus which causes AIDS, and which they call LAV-2.

AIDS and Europe

By January 1984 only 314 cases of AIDS had been seen in Europe, 88% of whom were males; the remaining 12% were mainly African females, and six children. The UK only had 31 cases at this time but by the end of 1986 nearly 600 cases had been reported. Initial analysis of at-risk populations in London showed that only 10% of seropositive individuals had developed AIDS[9] but cohort studies have now shown a steady rate of clinical deterioration in the rest of these patients. Studies of cohorts of HIV seropositive patients show that about 15% develop AIDS within 3 years. Five haemophiliacs who had documented dates of seroconversion took between 28 and 62 months to develop AIDS, clearly demonstrating the long latency between infection and clinical disease.

Computer programs predict that everyone who is infected will die of AIDS within 12 years. With at least 2 million people in the US and 30 000 people in the UK already infected the extent of the problem cannot be exaggerated.

PROSPECTS FOR TREATMENT

HIV is a retrovirus which critically depends on its reverse transcriptase (RT) to replicate. Studies on animal retroviruses have identified a number of RT inhibitors. Some of these were already in clinical use for other conditions but have now been tested against HIV *in vitro*. Suramin, phosphonoformate and azido thymidine (AZT) all show some RT inhibition, the latter being the most effective. Suramin is unfortunately too toxic to use. Recent trials with oral AZT have been encouraging although severe anaemia is a common side-effect. It seems likely that RT inhibitors would have to be given on a very long-term, or even lifelong basis, because the viral genome will remain within the host cell DNA.

Many other drugs have been reported as having a beneficial effect in AIDS including Ribavirin, isoprinosine, interferon and even Indocid and penicillamine. Ribavirin can inhibit RT *in vitro* but does not appear to have a significant effect *in vivo*. Isoprinosine is said to have both antiviral and immunostimulatory properties. The combination of Ribavirin and iso-prinosine is widely taken illegally in the US (as neither are prescribable there at present), and hence one of the largest drug trials in AIDS is not being monitored. Alpha interferon prevents HIV infection *in vitro* but has no effect *in vivo* although it may help in Kaposi's sarcoma. Gamma interferon appears to make KS worse.

Many new compounds will be offered for trial as anti-HIV agents over the next few years. It seems likely that a combination of an anti-viral and immunomodulating drug will eventually be the most effective. Even if an effective treatment is found, the need for a vaccine to protect individuals remains of paramount importance.

Vaccine development

The lack of neutralizing antibodies to HIV in infected individuals does not augur well for the development of an envelope vaccine. Nevertheless, a considerable effort has been put into this approach by many research groups. The envelope gene coding for gp110-120 has been cloned and expressed in vaccinia. Furthermore, peptides made from envelope sequences have been prepared and used to raise antibodies in a variety of animals. Unfortunately little neutralization is seen with these approaches, and even when weak neutralization is obtained it is usually only against the isolate from which the envelope antigens or peptides were prepared. This means that a traditional vaccine approach may take many years, especially as any vaccine will need to be tested in humans, since there is no suitable animal model.

Another approach is to prevent attachment of the virus to the CD4 antigen as this would 'neutralize' all known isolates. One way to achieve this is to inject antibodies against the CD4 antigen itself, but this might have serious effects on the immune system. Although mouse monoclonal antibodies against CD4 can be given to humans in the short term, not enough can be given to block all CD4 receptors. The better approach is to immunize with an anti-CD4 antibody, hoping that the patient will make anti-anti-CD4 (anti-idiotype) which will bind to the viral ligand and prevent its attachment to CD4+ lymphocytes. This approach is about to be tested in HIV-infected patients, and success will depend on their ability to produce high affinity anti-idiotype antibodies.

THE NEW VIRUSES

HTLV-IV, LAV-II

Retroviruses related to HIV have been isolated by Kanki and Essex from three putatively healthy Senegalese (HTLV-IV)[34] and by Clavel and colleagues[35] from two West African men with AIDS. These new viral isolates are morphologically similar to the classical HIV-I isolates. However, electron microscopy regularly shows spikes at the virion surface of these new isolates, which are not always observed in classical HIV. The *in vitro* cytopathic effects of LAV-II as compared to HIV-I isolates are essentially the same, whereas HTLV-IV is said not to cause cytopathic effects in primary culture but does form syncytia with CD4-positive cell lines.

The core antigens of these new viruses share some common epitopes with HIV-I. However, the envelope glycoproteins of HTLV-IV and LAV-II differ substantially from those of classical HIV. Interestingly, the envelope glycoprotein of LAV-II (gp140) is precipitated by sera from macaques infected with STLV-III; conversely LAV-II carriers produce antibodies which precipitate a protein of similar molecular weight from STLV-III virus extracts from macaques and wild-living African Green monkeys. These immunological cross-reactivities suggest that all these viruses have evolved from a common ancestor. However, hybridization experiments with HIV subgenomic probes have established the HTLV-IV and LAV-II are distantly related to HIV-I, and are distinct from the previously known simian retroviruses. The identification of HTLV-IV and LAV-II is extremely important for any further seroepidemiological studies, since both classical HIV-I and HTLV-IV/LAV-II antigens should be used.

HBLV

A human B cell-lymphotrophic virus (HBLV) was recently isolated from the peripheral blood leukocytes of six individuals[36,37]. Two were HIV-seropositive, one with AIDS-related lymphoma and one with dermatopathic lymphadenopathy. Of three HIV seronegative subjects living in the USA, one had angioimmunoblastic lymphadenopathy, one a cutaneous T-cell lymphoma and the other immunoblastic lymphoma. One HIV seronegative patient from Jamaica had a lymphocytic leukaemia. Antigenic analysis has revealed that all six isolates of HBLV are closely related. HBLV, which displays a specific affinity for freshly isolated human B lymphocytes, is a novel human herpes virus. It has a double-stranded DNA genome of greater than 110 kb pairs and is distinguishable from all known human and non-human primate herpes viruses by host range, *in vitro* biological effects, antigenic characteristics and structural features of viral genomic DNA. It is possible that HIV and HBLV are transmitted by similar modes so that a concomitant infection may occur. The oncogenic potential of HBLV is not known, but both the possible involvement of HBLV in the aetiology of various malignancies in AIDS patients and the possibility of 'just another opportunistic infection' should be considered. The same may apply for concomitant infections with HIV and HTLV-I.

References

1. Centers for Disease Control (1981). Kaposi's sarcoma and pneumocystis pneumonia among homosexual men - New York and California. *Morbid. Mortal. Weekly Rep.*, **30**, 305-8
2. Centers for Disease Control (1982). Epidemiological aspects of the current outbreak of Kaposi's sarcoma and opportunistic infections. *N. Engl. J. Med.*, **306**, 248-52
3. Lane, H. C. and Fauci, A. S. (1985). Immunological abnormalities in the acquired immunodeficiency syndrome. *Ann. Rev. Immunol.*, **3**, 477-500
4. Weiss, R. A. (1986). Supplement human T-cell retroviruses. In Weiss, R., Teich, N., Varmus, H. and Cottin, J. (eds.) *RNA Tumour Viruses: Molecular Biology of Tumor Viruses*. pp. 405-85. (New York: Cold Spring Harbor)
5. Gottlieb, M. S., Schroff, R., Schanker, H. M., Weisman, J. D., Fan, P. T., Wolf, R. A. and Saxon, A. (1981). *Pneumocystis carinii* pneumonia and mucosal candidiasis in previously healthy homosexual men. Evidence of a new acquired cellular immunodeficiency. *N. Engl. J. Med.*, **305**, 1425-31
6. Gottlieb, M. S., Groopman, J. E., Weinstein, W. M., Fahey, J. L. and Detels, R. (1983). The acquired immunodeficiency syndrome. *Ann. Intern. Med.*, **99**, 208-20
7. Centers for Disease Control (1982). Possible transfusion associated acquired immunodeficiency syndrome - California. *Morbid. Mortal. Weekly Rep.*, **31**, 652-4
8. Pinching, A. J. (1984). The acquired immunodeficiency syndrome. *Clin. Exp. Immunol.*, **56**, 1-13
9. Dalgleish, A. G. and Weiss, R. A. (1987). Human retroviruses. In Zuckerman, A., Bantavala and Pattison (eds.) *Clinical Virology*. pp. 517-44. (Chichester: Wiley and Sons)
10. Dalgleish, A. G. (1985). Human retroviruses. *Anat. N. Z. J. Med.*, **15**, 375-85
11. Gallo, R. C. (1984). Human T-cell leukaemia lymphoma virus and T-cell malignancies in adults. *Cancer Surveys*, **3**, 113-59
12. Hardy, W. D. (1985). Feline retroviruses. In Klein, G. (ed.) *Advances in Viral Oncology*. Vol 5, pp. 1-34. (New York: Raven Press)
13. Barre-Sinoussi, F., Chermann, F., Rey, F., Nugeyre, M. T., Chamaret, S., Gruest, J., Danguet, C., Axler-Blin, C., Vezinet-Brun, C., Rouzioux, C., Rozenbaum, W. and Montagner, L. (1983). Isolation of T-lymphotropic retrovirus from a patient at risk for acquired immunodeficiency syndrome (AIDS). *Science*, **220**, 868-70
14. Popovic, M., Sarngadharan, M. G., Read, E. and Gallo, R. C. (1984). A method for detection, isolation and continuous production of cytopathic human T-lymphotropic retroviruses of the HTLV family (HTLV-III) from patients with AIDS and pre-AIDS. *Science*, **224**, 497-500
15. Levy, J. A., Hoffman, A. D., Kramer, S. M., Landis, J. A., Shimabukuro, J. M. and Oshino, L. S. (1984). Isolation of lymphocytopathic retroviruses from San Francisco patients with AIDS. *Science*, **225**, 840-2
16. Wong Staal, F. and Gallo, R. C. (1985). Human T-lymphotropic retroviruses. *Nature*, **317**, 395-403
17. Cooper, D. A., Gold, J. and Maclean, P. (1985). Acute AIDS virus infection: definition of a clinical illness associated with seroconversion. *Lancet*, **1**, 537-40
18. Serwadda, D., Mugerwaum, R. D., Sewankaribo, N. K., Lwegaba, A., Carswell, J. W., Kirga, G. B., Bayley, A. C., Downing, R. G., Tedder, R. S., Clayden, S., Weiss, R. A. and Dalgleish, A. G. (1985). Slim disease: a new disease in Uganda and its association with HTLV-III infection. *Lancet*, **2**, 849-52
19. Costello, C., Treacy, M. and Lai, L. (1986). Treatment of immune trombocytopenic purpura in homosexual men. *Scand. J. Haematol.*, **36**, 507-10.
20. Berger, J. R. and Resnick, L. (1987). HTLV-III/LAV-related neurological disease In Broder, S. (ed.) AIDS - Modern Concepts and Therapeutic Challenges pp. 263-83. (New York: Dekker)
21. Dalgleish, A. G. and McElwain, T. (1986). A viral aetiology for Hodgkins disease. *Aust. N.Z. J. Med.*, **16**, 823-7.
22. Marshall, C. J. (1985). Human oncogenes. In Weiss, R. A., Teich, N., Varmus, H. and Coffin, J. (eds.) *RNA Tumour Viruses*. Vol. 2. pp. 487-558 (New York: Cold Spring Harbor Laboratories)
23. Dalgleish, A. G. (1986). The T4 molecule: function and structure. *Immunol. Today*, **7**, 142-4

24. Dalgleish, A. G. (1986). Antiviral strategies and vaccines against HTLV III/LAV. *J. R. Coll. Phys.*, **20**, 258–67
25. Hoxie, J. A. *et al.* (1985). Persistent non-cytopathic infection of normal human T lymphocytes with AIDS-associated retrovirus. *Science*, **229**, 1400–2
26. Walker, C. M., Moody, D. J., Stites, D. P. and Levy, J. A. (1986). CD8+ lymphocytes can control HIV infection *in vitro* by suppressing virus replication. *Science*, **234**, 1563–6
27. Laurence, J. and Mayer, L. (1984). Immunoregulatory lymphokines of T hybridomas from AIDS patients: constitutive and inducible suppressor factors. *Science*, **225**, 66–9
28. Malkovsky, M. *et al.* (1982). Non-specific inhibitor released by T acceptor cells reduces the production of interleakin-2. *Nature (London)*, **300**, 652–5
29. Schnittman, S. M. *et al.* (1986). Direct polyclonal activation of human B lymphocytes by the acquired immune deficiency syndrome virus. *Science*, **233**, 1084–6
30. Desai, S. M., Kalyanaraman, V. S., Cassey, J. M., Srinivasan, A., Andersen P. R. and Devare, S. G. (1986). Molecular cloning and primary nucleotide sequence analysis of a distinct human immunodeficiency virus isolate reveal significant divergence in its genomic sequences, *Proc. Natl. Acad. Sci. USA*, **83**, 8380–4
31. Sodroski, J., Goh, W. C., Rosen, C., Dayton, A., Terrwilliger, E. and Haseltine, W. (1986). A second post transcriptional trans activator gene required for HTLV-III replication. *Nature (London)*, **321**, 412–17
32. Bayley, A. C., Downing, R. G., Popov, R. C., Tedder, R. S., Dalgleish, A. G. and Weiss, R. A. (1985). HTLV III distinguishes between atypical and endemic Kaposi's sarcoma in Africa. *Lancet*, **1**, 359–61
33. Biggar, R. J. (1986). The AIDS problem in Africa. *Lancet*, **1**, 79–82
34. Kanki, P. J., Barin, F., M'Boup, S., Allan, J. S., Lemone, J. L. R., Marlink, R., McClane, M., Lee, T. H., Arbeille, B., Dennis, F. and Essex, M. (1986). New human T-lymphotropic retrovirus related to Simian T-lymphotropic virus type III (STLV-III AGM). *Science*, **232**, 238–43
35. Clavel, F., Guetard, D., Brun Vezinet, F., Chamanet, S., Rey, M. A., Santos Ferreira, S., Laurent, A. G., Dauguet, C., Katlama, C., Rouzioux, C., Klatzmann, D., Champalimaud, J. C. and Montagnier, J. C. (1986). Isolation of a new human retrovirus from West African patients with AIDS. *Science*, **233**, 343–6
36 Salahuddin, S. Z., Ablashi, D., Markham, P., Josephs, S., Sturzenegger, S. F., Kaplan, M., Halligan, G., Biberfield, P., Wong-Staal, F., Kramarsky, B. and Gallo, R. C. (1986). Isolation of a new virus, HBLV, in patients with lymphoproliferative disorders. *Science*, **234**, 596–601
37. Josephs, S. F., Salahuddin, S. Z., Ablashi, D. V., Schachter, F., Wong-Staal, F. and Gallo, R. C. (1986). Genomic analysis of the human B-lymphotropic virus (HBLV). *Science*, **234**, 601–3

2
Hypogammaglobulinaemia: Recent Advances

A. D. B. WEBSTER AND G. P. SPICKETT

INTRODUCTION

Soon after the technology for serum protein electrophoresis became available, Bruton was able to diagnose a child with hypogammaglobulinaemia who probably had acquired disease rather than the inherited X-linked variety[1]. Janeway et al.[2] described more cases a few years later, showing that adults can also be affected. The Medical Research Council's survey in the 1960s showed that the majority of patients in the UK acquired the disease as adults[3]. A rough estimate at present is that there are about 500 patients with 'primary' non-familial hypogammaglobulinaemia in the UK population of approximately 55 million, with about 50 males having definite X-linked disease. The term 'primary' is taken to mean that the hypogammaglobulinaemia is not associated with a lymphoid malignancy (e.g. chronic lymphatic leukaemia, myeloma) or has been induced by drugs. However, this terminology is likely to be superseded by a more descriptive classification (see Table 2.1). Selective deficiencies of IgG subclasses and of IgA are discussed in Chapter 5. Some patients with selective deficiencies of both IgA and IgG$_2$ may be included under the broad classification of 'primary' hypogammaglobulinaemia if the total serum IgG is low. These distinctions are at present academic, as it is likely that there is a spectrum of severity of non-familial (acquired) hypogammaglobulinaemia, ranging from selective IgA deficiency through a combination of IgA and IgG subclass deficiencies, to severe panhypogammaglobulinaemia. It is easy to recognize the latter clinically, and consequently patients in this severe end of the spectrum will be discussed here in some detail.

Most immunologists believe that primary non-familial hypogammaglobulinaemia is a syndrome with many different aetiologies. Clearly one can separate those very rare patients with rubella- or Epstein-Barr virus-induced immunodeficiency, and there is good reason to believe that hypogammaglobulinaemia associated with thymoma is a separate entity. However, opinions

Table 2.1 Hypogammaglobulinaemia

---

(1) *X-linked*

    (a) severe (agammaglobulinaemia)
    (b) moderate (usually in male siblings)
    (c) with high serum IgM

    X-linked lymphoproliferative syndrome (EB virus associated)

(2) *Primary - non-familial (common variable)*

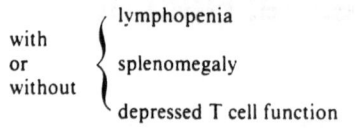

with
or
without
   lymphopenia
   splenomegaly
   depressed T cell function

    with thymoma (adults over 40 years)

(3) *Secondary*

    Virus-related

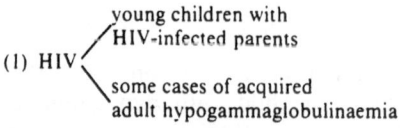

    (1) HIV
       young children with HIV-infected parents
       some cases of acquired adult hypogammaglobulinaemia

    (2) Rubella – rare in children with rubella syndrome

    Drugs
    Phenytoin
    Gold
    Penicillamine
    Sulphasalazine
    Cytotoxics/steroids (uncommon)

    'Malignant' B cell disorders
    Chronic lymphatic leukaemia
    Myeloma

    Increased loss of immunoglobulin
    Nephrotic syndrome
    Intestinal lymphangiectasia
    Other protein-losing enteropathies

---

differ as to whether the mechanism of the hypogammaglobulinaemia is similar in the majority of patients and that the variable T cell abnormalities are para-phenomena. Most physicians call this disease 'common variable' hypogammaglobulinaemia (CVH).

X-LINKED AGAMMAGLOBULINAEMIA

There are probably three different types of X-linked disease, possibly due to different mutations of a gene on the X chromosome. The classic type is characterized by a clear family history involving at least two generations, severe infections within the first 2 years of life and virtually unrecordable serum immunoglobulins. These children usually develop bronchiectasis before adolescence and are particularly prone to echovirus and mycoplasma infections[4]. The second type is less severe, the serum IgG being measurable, often over 0.1 g/l, and the patients tending to have much milder chest disease. In our experience this milder type has occurred in families where all the male siblings of a single generation are affected, implying a new mutation in the mothers, with possibly some selective advantage for the abnormal X chromosome during meiosis to explain why all male siblings are affected.

The third type is where IgM production is retained, the patients sometimes having very high serum IgM levels[5]. It is not clear whether this condition is really the X-linked lymphoproliferative syndrome (XLPS) with a particularly severe depression of IgG and IgA synthesis. At all events, such patients are very rare, and we are not aware of any families in the south of England with this condition, other than those associated with XLPS.

INFECTIONS (TABLE 2.2)

Patients with all types of hypogammaglobulinaemia are prone to recurrent upper and lower respiratory tract infections, usually with non-typable *Haemophilus influenzae*, but also with mycoplasma species and pneumococci. Unless adequately treated, bronchiectasis is a common sequela. Chronic middle ear sepsis is common in affected children and should be energetically treated to avoid permanent hearing loss. The management of these common infections has been adequately reviewed elsewhere[4]. However, it is appropriate to briefly highlight recent developments in the management of echovirus and mycoplasma infections.

Echovirus infection

Although this can occur in patients with acquired hypogammaglobulinaemia, it is much more common in those with X-linked disease[6]. The complete lack of antibody in the severe form of X-linked agammaglobulinaemia appears to be the major predisposing factor for chronic echovirus infection of the central nervous system and muscles. These echoviruses, of which there are 34 serotypes, cause a chronic vasculitis affecting the meninges of the brain and

Table 2.2 Infections in hypogammaglobulinaemic patients

	Common	*Rare*
Respiratory tract	*Haemophilus influenzae* (non-encapsulated) Pneumococci	Atypical mycobacteria *Branhamella catarrhalis*
Gastrointestinal tract	Campylobacters *Giardia lamblia*	Cryptosporidium Salmonella
Urinary tract	Ureaplasmas	
Central nervous system	echovirus pneumococci	
Skin/mucous membranes	*Herpes zoster*	*Candida albicans*

spinal cord, the muscles and occasionally the small vessels in the subcutaneous tissues of the extremities. The muscles gradually become fibrotic, producing contractures and a characteristic posture due to flexion of the elbows and knees. Chronic inflammation and thickening of the meninges occurs in the central nervous system, with frequent involvement of the 8th nerve and deafness, recurrent convulsions, headache and finally death due to involvement of vital centres in the brainstem. Patients may survive with the disease for as long as 8 years, showing a gradual but relentless deterioration. Echovirus can be isolated from the cerebral spinal fluid, and sometimes the muscles, even in the early stages of the disease when there are no central nervous system signs. Sometimes a different serotype is isolated from CSF and muscle; it is not clear whether this is due to a mutation in the original virus or infection with two separate strains.

There have been numerous attempts to treat these patients with specific antibodies to the relevant echovirus serotype, either using hyperimmune animal serum, or human plasma from hyperimmune donors. Some patients have been given batches of intravenous gammaglobulin which contain a relatively high antibody titre to the virus. There is a strong clinical impression that such therapy can alleviate symptoms and retard the progression of the disease, but nearly all cases have relapsed when the treatment is discontinued. Permanent cures may have occurred in one Polish patient who received intravenous gammaglobulin[7], and another patient in the USA who was given intrathecal gammaglobulin via an Omaha reservoir[8]. Echovirus disease is now very rare in the UK, possibly because most patients with X-linked agammaglobulinaemia now receive regular intravenous gammaglobulin which may contain enough protective antibody.

Mycoplasma infection

Mycoplasma pneumoniae, but also 'non-pathogenic' commensal strains such as *M. hominis*, *M. salivarium* and *Ureaplasma urealyticum* can cause serious chronic infection in hypogammaglobulinaemic patients[9]. As in immuno-competent patients, *M. pneumoniae* can cause chronic low grade pneumonia, and should be considered in hypogammaglobulinaemic patients who do not improve on co-trimoxazole or ampicillin. *U. urealyticum* is a common 'commensal' in the female urogenital tract and is also a recognized cause of urethritis in men[10]. Patients with X-linked agammaglobulinaemia are particularly prone to ureaplasma urethritis and cystitis, the organisms then seeding to joints. *In vitro* studies have shown that mycoplasmas are phagocytosed by neutrophils in the absence of antibody, either directly via receptors on the neutrophil surface or through activation of the classical complement pathway, and then via complement receptors[11]. However, the organisms remain viable inside neutrophils which presumably carry them to joints via the bloodstream. In contrast, specific antibodies inhibit the growth of mycoplasmas *in vitro*, supporting the clinical impression that they are critical for host defence against these organisms.

The diagnosis should be suspected if the joint aspirate is purulent and no bacteria are seen with the Gram stain. The fluid should be cultured for standard pathogens such as *H. influenzae*, pneumococci or staphylococci, but the patients should be immediately treated with high dose intravenous tetracycline and erythromycin because mycoplasmas are the commonest cause of septic arthritis in hypogammaglobulinaemic patients in the United Kingdom. Most mycoplasmas are sensitive to these drugs, but injections of hyperimmune animal serum may have to be considered if the organism is resistant[12]. Patients should be warned to report the first signs of urethritis or cystitis, when they should be treated empirically with oral doxycycline until the diagnosis can be confirmed. It should be remembered that most routine laboratories cannot isolate mycoplasmas, and usually depend upon serology for the diagnosis of *M. pneumoniae*. This is obviously inappropriate in antibody deficient patients, so that swabs and aspirates have to be sent to special supra-regional laboratories for culture

GAMMAGLOBULIN REPLACEMENT THERAPY

It is not our intention to extensively review this important subject here, but it is appropriate to highlight some recent advances. Nearly all hypogammaglobulinaemic patients worldwide were treated with regular intramuscular gammaglobulin injections up until the late 1970s, although some clinics used fresh frozen plasma infusions. Because of the risk of AIDS and non-A non-B hepatitis, the latter has been abandoned in most countries. There is general agreement that only about a third of hypogammaglobulinaemic patients are adequately protected against infections by intramuscular gammaglobulin, and although the rest show improvement they remain prone to *H. influenzae*, mycoplasma and echovirus infections[13]. Although some of the early intravenous gammaglobulin (IVIG) preparations transmitted non-A non-B hepatitis, there is now evidence that most of the currently available preparations are safe[14]. Patients usually improve when their treatment is switched from intramuscular to intravenous therapy, and there is a strong clinical impression that the latter is needed to prevent bronchiectasis in children with X-linked agammaglobulinaemia. Furthermore, high dose IVIG $(0.6\,g\,kg^{-1}\,month^{-1})$ can produce a significant improvement in lung function in those with parenchymal damage[15]. Our current policy is to treat all hypogammaglobulinaemic patients with evidence of bronchiectasis, severe chronic sinusitis or middle ear disease with fortnightly intravenous gammaglobulin at a dose of 200 mg/kg body weight. Although there is very little antibody to either echovirus or mycoplasmas in these preparations, it is interesting that we have not seen these infections in any patient regularly treated with IVIG. Most patients are very impressed with the improvement after starting intravenous therapy, and many in the USA and UK have now been trained to give their own infusions at home.

THE AETIOLOGY OF HYPOGAMMAGLOBULINAEMIA

X-linked

Frøland and Natvig (1972)[16] were two of the first to show that patients with X-linked agammaglobulinaemia lacked circulating lymphocytes with surface

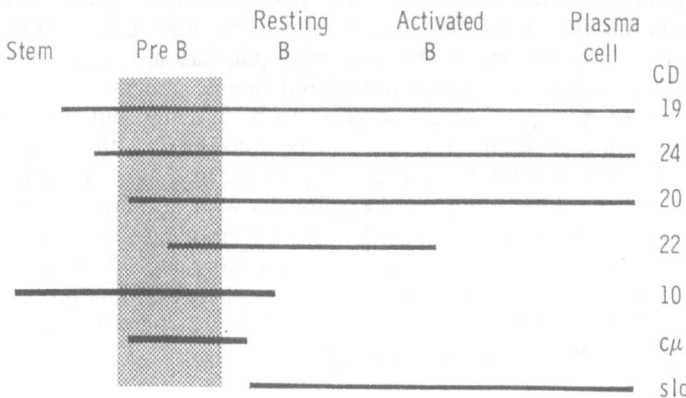

Figure 2.1 Diagram showing markers which recognize various stages of B cell ontogeny (solid lines). CD 10-24 are differentiation antigens recognized by monoclonal antibodies. $C\mu$ = cytoplasmic IgM; SIg = surface immunoglobulin (IgM). The hatched area denotes site of 'block' in X-linked agammaglobulinaemia

immunoglobulin (SIg). At the time this was thought to be pathognomic, but then patients with non-familial hypogammaglobulinaemia were described without circulating SIg[+] lymphocytes. The recent availability of a variety of monoclonal antibodies to B cell differentiation antigens has permitted more precise localization of the defect[17]. There appears to be a block in B cell differentiation at a stage when the cells leave the bone marrow, and after immunoglobulin gene rearrangement occurs. Pre-B cells[18], recognized by their cytoplasmic IgM, and an excess of CD10 (CALLA) positive cells can be found in the bone marrows of patients with X-linked agammaglobulinaemia, and the latter may 'spill over' into the circulation (Figure 2.1).

Two groups of geneticists in the USA have recently demonstrated that the defect lies within the B cell, and not in some other cell which produces a B-cell differentiating factor[19, 20]. Both groups have shown that all the circulating B cells in healthy obligate heterozygote mothers carry an active normal X chromosome, implying that those B cells carrying the active abnormal chromosome have failed to mature. The Lyon hypothesis of random X chromosome inactivation during embryogenesis dictates that this is not possible unless the defect is intrinsic to the B cell. Heterozygote females with suitable polymorphic genetic markers for such studies can therefore be recognized by using such sophisticated techniques, although these are too complicated at present for routine use.

There is no evidence that cellular immunity is significantly compromised in patients with XLA; for instance the circulating T lymphocyte count is normal and delayed hypersensitivity skin reactivity is intact. However, their circulating T cells have an 'immature' phenotype, as shown by a fetal lactate dehydrogenase (cytoplasmic) isoenzyme pattern[21] and a low activity of ecto 5'-nucleotidase (5'N) (plasma membrane)[22]. Their circulating monocytes also have very low ecto-5'N activity which rises to normal after overnight

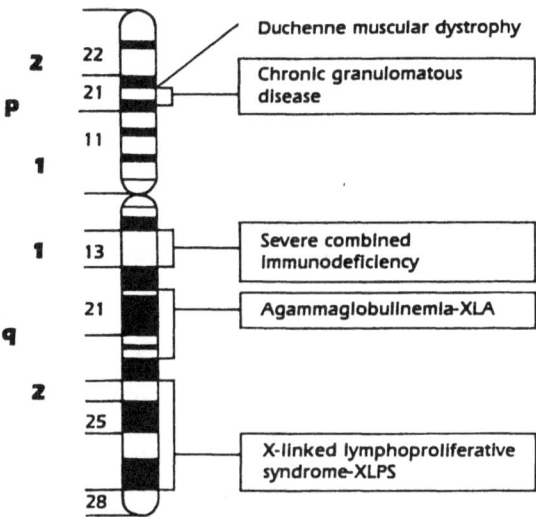

Figure 2.2 Localization of the genetic defects in the X-chromosome causing immunodeficiency

incubation *in vitro* (Webster and Bird, unpublished). One explanation for these abnormalities is an increased turnover of lymphocytes and monocytes, although this is unlikely to be due to infection since such changes do not occur in immunocompetent patients with bronchitis or pneumonia. It is more likely that antibody or immune complexes directly or indirectly stimulate T cells and monocytes to mature.

Another potentially confusing aspect of T cell function in XLA is the finding that the circulating lymphocytes from some patients, particularly those with clinically more severe disease (Type 1), have excessive suppressor activity for *in vitro* immunoglobulin production when mixed with B cells from normal donors[23, 24]. This is apparently not related to intravenous gammaglobulin therapy, despite claims of such an effect, and is probably indirectly related to chronic infection. Similar T cell abnormalities occur in about 10% of CVH patients (see below). The finding that XLA T cells may suppress the B cells from only some normal donors suggests that the mechanism involves MHC Class II antigens[24].

The X-chromosome

Using DNA probes for restriction fragment length polymorphisms (RFLPs) on the X-chromosome, it is possible to show a close linkage with the 19.2 and S21 probes in most patients[25, 26]. This localizes the defective gene to the Xq21–22 area on the proximal segment of the long arm (Figure 2.2). Providing there are enough members in at least two generations of an XLA family for study, there is a very good chance of recognizing the female carriers[27]. Such studies are likely to help localize the XLA gene more precisely in the next few years, hopefully leading to cloning of the gene itself whose product is likely to be of great interest to immunologists. As with many other genetic diseases (e.g. thalassaemia), a number of different mutations within the DXS17 region are likely to cause XLA[26].

Genetic counselling

As discussed above, there are time consuming methods for identifying female carriers, but there are no routine facilities for doing this yet in the UK. Analysis of B cell populations in fetal blood at 16 weeks cannot provide a definitive diagnosis, unlike the diagnostic changes in T cell subpopulations in a fetus with severe combined immunodeficiency[28]. However, probes for RFLPs closely linked to the XLA gene can theoretically now be used on DNA obtained from chorionic villus biopsies with only a small chance of error. Nevertheless, early diagnosis after the birth of a male infant in affected families remains crucial. If there are no circulatory SIg⁺ B cells in the newborn, then prophylactic intramuscular gammaglobulin should be given weekly. By 3 months, most of the maternal IgG will have disappeared and the diagnosis can be confirmed by the presence of severe hypogammaglobulinaemia and persistent absence of circulating 'mature' B cells.

X-LINKED LYMPHOPROLIFERATIVE SYNDROME (DUNCAN'S SYNDROME)

XLPS was first described some 12 years ago in males of the Duncan family who had an inherited disorder characterized by immunodeficiency with frequently fatal infectious mononucleosis. Survivors had a chronic EBV infection often accompanied by profound hypogammaglobulinaemia and an increased incidence of lymphoma[29]. Up until the primary infection with EBV, the susceptible males are normal. Family studies have confirmed the X-linked transmission of the condition.

When normal people are infected with EBV, a well-described series of immunological events takes place, characterized by the appearance of a lymphocytosis and antibodies to the early antigen (EA) and viral capsid antigen (VCA). The former are transitory but the latter persist. EBV-specific cytotoxic cells appear and lyse infected cells; this releases the EBV nuclear antigen (EBNA), and antibodies to this may then be detected. Latent infections may be reactivated by immunosuppression, and in these cases there is a rise in the VCA titre, a drop in the EBNA titre and the reappearance of EA antibodies. Patients with XLPS show a similar pattern, and female carriers also have elevated anti-VCA and anti-EA titres[30].

Numerous functional defects have been described (reviewed by Hanto et al.[31]). A fundamental defect has been thought to be failure of T cells to recognize and kill EBV-infected B cells, allowing unchecked proliferation. In vitro antibody production is impaired and this correlates with the occurrence of hypogammaglobulinaemia; it is suggested that this is directly related to the EBV infection of the B cells, but we have preliminary evidence in a single patient that the defect includes a failure to provide specific help by T cells, and that the effect is most marked for IgG (Spickett, unpublished). However, the T cells and dendritic cells from this patient induced excessive IgM production from normal B cells when stimulated with PWM, while stimulating no IgG. The rarity of such patients means that it is difficult to study large numbers. Other reported defects include decreased memory T cell activity against EBV, and impaired NK cell activity, which may have relevance to the development of lymphomas due to reduced immune surveillance to which NK cells are known to contribute[32].

Recent molecular genetic studies on an extensive XLPS family have allowed the detection of a marker restriction fragment length polymorphism which co-segregates with the, as yet unknown, XLPS locus on the X-chromosome[33]. This marker will permit the detection of carrier females and the prenatal diagnosis of affected males. Hopefully, identification of the relevant gene(s) and its function in immune regulation should follow rapidly.

'COMMON VARIABLE' HYPOGAMMAGLOBULINAEMIA (CVH)

Clinical features

Affected patients suffer from the same types of infection as those with X-linked agammaglobulinaemia, although echovirus and mycoplasma infections are less common in this group. About a third of patients have splenomegaly, which in some cases may be massive causing hypersplenism with neutropenia and thrombocytopenia. Chronic gastritis, achlorhydria and a high incidence of gastric carcinoma[34], as well as autoimmune blood dyscrasias[35] are features which occur in CVH patients but not in those with X-linked disease.

Genetic factors

There is very little evidence of a genetic predisposition to CVH. However, a minority of patients have first-degree relatives with selective IgA deficiency, and overall there is a slightly increased incidence of autoantibodies to thyroid and stomach in first-degree relatives[36]. This does not necessarily imply the presence of genetic factors, and could just as well be explained by transmission of a lymphotropic virus in these families. There are a few intriguing families where a parent, either the mother or father, and a child are affected[37]. The disease occurs worldwide but the only proper attempt to estimate prevalence was done in the 1960s in the United Kingdom[3].

Immunology (Table 2.3)

In contrast to patients with X-linked agammaglobulinaemia, about 50% of those with CVH are lymphopenic, and in some this may predominantly involve the T4 lymphocytes causing a reversed T4/T8 ratio. Lymphopenia is more common in those patients with splenomegaly, and those patients with lymphopenia are more likely to be anergic to a variety of delayed hypersensitivity skin test antigens and to show poor *in vitro* lymphocyte transformation to mitogens[38].

Table 2.3 Circulating lymphocyte defects in acquired hypogammaglobulinaemia

---

T cells

Low activity of
(a) α-naphthyl esterase*
(b) ecto 5'-nucleotidase* (abnormal K_m)
(c) malate and lactate dehydrogenase (fetal LDH isoenzyme pattern)*
(d) dipeptidyl peptidase IV (high K_m)

Poor *in vitro* proliferation with mitogens (30% of patients)

Depressed 'Help'*
⎤
⎟⎟ for Ig production in PWM
'Increased suppression' ⎟ driven systems
(only 10% of patients) ⎦

Antigen presenting (dendritic) cells
Depressed PWM presentation for *in vitro* Ig production

B cells
Variable numbers in circulation*
Normal EBV-induced *in vitro* IgM production (low IgG)*
Low *in vitro* IgG production in PWM driven systems*

---

*compatible with a block in the maturation of lymphocytes by comparison with cord blood cells

In 1974, Waldmann *et al.*[39] described a patient whose T lymphocytes suppressed *in vitro* pokeweed-induced immunoglobulin (Ig) production by normal B cells. It was initially thought that this might explain the hypogammaglobulinaemia, but subsequently it became clear that only a small subset (about 15%) of patients had excess suppressor T cells in their circulation[40]. Although it is possible that this might exacerbate the immunodeficiency, it is now generally considered to be a secondary phenomenon. However, the induction of these T suppressor cells is not understood, but could be due to a chronic viral infection or even to gammaglobulin replacement therapy. It may be relevant that haemophiliacs receiving factor VIII develop a relative increase in circulating T8 cells, not apparently related to contracting non-A non-B hepatitis or HIV infection[41].

T helper function

The T cells from CVH patients show normal help for *in vitro* Ig production when mixed with normal B cells in a pokeweed stimulated system[42]. Furthermore, they will provide help in an antigen specific driven system if the T cells are obtained from tetanus toxoid (TT) immunized CVH patients and then added to normal B cells in the presence of TT[43]. However, T cell help for Ig production is depressed in the majority of CVH patients in a more sensitive system when normal dendritic cells are pulsed with pokeweed and then added to normal B cells and the patient's irradiated T cells[24]. The finding of a consistent functional defect in T cells complements other enzymatic abnormalities which will now be briefly discussed

Lymphocyte enzyme abnormalities

The original serendipidous observation that the circulating lymphocytes of CVH patients had very low activity of the lymphocyte plasma membrane enzyme, ecto 5'-nucleotidase (5'N) has been confirmed by many workers[22, 44]. Furthermore, it is clear that the T cells have low activity, which cannot be explained by abnormalities in the ratio of different T cell subsets using currently available markers[45]. The physiological function of 5'N is not understood, but it probably has a role in salvaging extracellular nucleotides (e.g. adenosine monophosphate) to supplement intracellular purine stores. This might be particularly useful for rapidly dividing cells such as lymphocytes. However, inhibiting the enzyme *in vitro* does not depress lymphocyte transformation or pokeweed mitogen-induced immunoglobulin production[46]. Nevertheless, repeated injections of the 5'N inhibitor (AOPCP) into mice did inhibit the *in vivo* primary antibody response to sheep red blood cells[47]. Thus, there is some evidence that 5'N is involved in the immune response and might be more directly linked with the antibody deficiency in CVH patients.

The low activity of lymphocyte 5'N in CVH patients is due to altered kinetics of the enzyme which requires a much higher concentration of the substrate, AMP, to function[48]. Three other T lymphocyte ecto enzymes have been investigated: adenosine diphosphatase, γ-glutamyl transferase and dipeptidyl peptidase IV, but only the latter is abnormal, having a lower K_m than normal (Shah *et al.*, unpublished). These changes may reflect an increase in the numbers of immature lymphocytes in the circulation, perhaps due to increased turnover, a view which is supported by the fact that lymphocyte 5'N activity is low in cord blood. However, there are other lymphocyte enzyme defects in CVH which are not compatible with this hypothesis, and which suggest a more generalized metabolic defect (Table 2.3). In this context it is interesting that the circulating lymphocytes from patients with AIDS have low 5'N activity, although only a minority of cells are infected with HIV. An understanding of the mechanism of this defect may throw light on the aetiology of CVH where a retrovirus may also be implicated (see below).

Antigen-presenting cells

Two different systems have been used to analyse antigen-presenting cells in CVH patients. In the first, monocytes are pulsed with *E. coli* antigen, and the proliferation of autologous T cells measured[49]. The majority of CVH patients show a depressed response in this system but this may be non-specific since early studies showed that many patients have poor T cell proliferation with mitogens[38, 50]. The pulsed monocytes from only one out of three CVH patients failed to stimulate T cells from a healthy HLA identical relative, suggesting that there was nothing intrinsically abnormal in the monocytes from most patients. In contrast, pokeweed pulsed circulating antigen presenting (dendritic) cells from CVH patients stimulate very little immunoglobulin from normal B and T cell mixtures when compared to dendritic cells from normal donors, and will even suppress the function of normal dendritic cells.

All six CVH patients studied showed this defect, in contrast to normal activity with the cells from patients with X-linked agammaglobulinaemia[24]. The latter is an important 'positive' control because it shows that lack of antibody, or immunoglobulin replacement therapy, does not induce these defects.

B cells

The number of circulating B cells is very variable, with about a third of CVH patients having no SIg-positive B cells, although occasionally immature forms recognized by monoclonal markers are present. The majority of circulating B cells in the rest are SIgM positive[51]. This probably explains why EBV-induced B cell clones from these patients secrete near normal amounts of IgM *in vitro* with very little IgG and IgA[52]. The overall picture is compatible with a failure of B cell maturation beyond the stage of IgM production.

THYMOMA WITH HYPOGAMMAGLOBULINAEMIA

This condition occurs in adults over 40 years of age. The thymoma is usually a benign and well encapsulated spindle cell tumour, its removal having no effect on the hypogammaglobulinaemia[53]. Affected patients have a tendency to opportunistic infections, particularly candidiasis, and are also prone to autoimmune blood dyscrasias. Most patients lack SIg-positive circulating B cells and frequently have an excess of suppressor T cells in the circulation which inhibit *in vitro* Ig synthesis by pokeweed-stimulated normal B cells. Pre-B cells were absent in all of three patients investigated by Hayward *et al.* and their circulating T cells suppressed the *in vitro* formation of pre-B cells in normal bone marrows[54]. However, a patient has been described with circulating SIg+ B cells without suppressor T cells, suggesting that the reduced Ig levels cannot be attributed solely to the presence of suppressor phenomena and/or a block in early B cell differentiation[55].

SECONDARY HYPOGAMMAGLOBULINAEMIA

This section discusses the aetiological relationship of some viruses, drugs and clonal B cell disorders with antibody deficiency. Secondary hypogammaglobulinaemia due to excessive loss of gammaglobulin (e.g. protein losing enteropathy) is not discussed. The hypogammaglobulinaemia in this situation is usually mild and not associated with severe infections.

Viruses and hypogammaglobulinaemia

Rubella virus

Rubella virus has long been recognized as a rare cause of hypogammaglobulinaemia, usually causing a low serum IgG and IgA, often with a raised IgM, in a minority of young children with congenital rubella syndrome. No significant work has been done on this association recently, and with the rapid decline in the prevalence of this condition it is unlikely that further studies will be feasible.

Cytomegalovirus (CMV)

Cytomegalovirus occasionally appears in classifications of immuno-deficiency, but there is little evidence that it causes hypogamma-globulinaemia. However, animal models of CMV infection have demon-strated depressed antibody production, reduced γ-IFN production and poor mitogen responsiveness. Infected mice have a reduced capacity to clear bacteria, which appears to involve not only antibody deficiency but also a failure of neutrophil phagocytosis[56]. In normal humans reduced T cell reactivity to mitogens and other viruses has been documented, accompanied by a reduction in the CD4$^+$ cells and a reversal of the CD4/CD8 ratio[57]. Interestingly, a reduction of CMV-specific lymphocyte proliferation has been found in pregnant women, which may be of importance in determining the outcome of CMV infection in pregnancy and the effect on the fetus[58]. As a rule, the earlier in life infection occurs the more profound the immunosuppression.

Retroviruses

Most HIV-infected patients have hypergammaglobulinaemia, but their specific antibody responses are poor, and may be absent in the terminal phase of the disease[59]. This dichotomy between excessive production of immuno-globulins and depressed specific antibody responses has not been explained, although there are claims that HIV-1 directly stimulates B lymphocytes *in vitro* (polyclonal activation)[60]. The picture is further confused by reports of HIV-infected infants and young children who are hypogammaglobulinaemic, a finding of practical diagnostic importance since these patients are seronegative for HIV[61].

The isolation of retroviruses from two CVH patients without any risk factors for AIDS suggest that we still have a lot to learn about the transmission and origin of the human HIVs[62]. The viruses were closely related to HIV-1, and one of the patients died from opportunistic infections. Attempts to isolate retroviruses from a further 42 CVH patients have been disappointing, although there was evidence of infection in two[63]. If CVH is a retroviral disease, then the infection must be partially controlled or confined to a subpopulation of cells in the majority of patients. The concept of acquired hypogammaglobulinaemia being a retroviral disease is appealing since there is a large family of HIV-related retroviruses which cause disease in animals, some of them remaining 'latent' in the immune system for long periods[64].

Drugs and hypogammaglobulinaemia

Immunosuppressive agents, particularly cyclophosphamide and azathioprine, occasionally induce hypogammaglobulinaemia after prolonged treatment. It is likely that many more patients on these and other cytotoxic drugs have a significant functional impairment of antibody production despite normal serum immunoglobulin levels, although this is rarely tested. There is a growing number of drugs which unexpectedly cause hypogamma-globulinaemia in a small percentage of patients (Table 2.1). It is therefore important to take a careful history of drug treatment to avoid diagnosing CVH incorrectly. The hypogammaglobulinaemia may persist for some years after stopping the drug, although usually there is a steady rise in the immunoglobulin levels within a few months. Apart from the recognized immunosuppressive agents, it is not known how these other drugs affect the immune system.

Chronic lymphatic leukaemia (CLL)

It has been apparent for some years that infection, mainly bacterial, is a major problem in most CLL patients. The role of immunodeficiency in this predisposition has been reviewed recently by Chapel and Bunch[65]. Briefly, the major correlate of increased infection is concomitant hypogamma-globulinaemia. Specific immunization demonstrates poor primary and secondary responses to a variety of antigens. Trials are currently in progress to assess the effectiveness of intravenous gammaglobulin in reducing infective episodes. Virus infections are rare, and defects in T cell-mediated immune responses are more likely to be caused by chemotherapy than by the underlying disease. Neutrophil function is likewise only impaired in patients aggressively treated with chemotherapy. There is presently no evidence for defects in the complement system, and the increased incidence of pneumococcal infection, together with poor opsonization reported in some patients, is most probably due to lack of specific antibody.

The mechanism for the antibody deficiency is unclear. The best explanation is that the lymphoid architecture of the spleen and lymph nodes becomes so distorted by the presence of the malignant clone that the necessary cellular interactions for antibody production cannot occur. There may be other factors since there is a poor correlation between the extent of the clonal B cell infiltration and the immunodeficiency.

Multiple myeloma

Patients with multiple myeloma are at increased risk of bacterial infections. Most patients with malignant paraproteinaemias have significantly reduced polyclonal immunoglobulins, and as a result have reduced responsiveness to challenge with antigens such as pneumococcal polysaccharides, and their B cells show poor immunoglobulin production *in vitro* when stimulated with pokeweed mitogen[66]. This contrasts with the normal humoral responses seen in patients with benign monoclonal gammopathies. The cause of the reduced responses is unclear. Suppression of B cell function by monocytes has been demonstrated in patients, and a similar phenomenon occurs in experimental myeloma in mice. However, a secondary effect due to cytotoxic therapy may explain these abnormalities in humans since studies in untreated patients have not confirmed these findings. However, it is clear that there is a primary defect at the level of the B cell *in vitro*, and that in most patients T cell function is normal. There are substantial numbers of B cells derived from the malignant clone in the circulation and bone marrow of patients with myeloma, and these are probably responsible for preventing normal B cells making, immunoglobulin bearing the same light chain on the malignant clone.

References

1. Bruton, O. C. (1952). Agammaglobulinaemia. *Pediatrics*, **9**, 722
2. Janeway, C. A., Apt, L. and Gitlin, D. (1953). Agammaglobulinaemia. *Trans. Assoc. Am. Phys.*, **66**, 200
3. Hill, L. E. (1971). Clinical features of hypogammaglobulinaemia. In *Hypogammaglobulinaemia in the United Kingdom*. Medical Research Council Series SRS 310, p. 9
4. Asherson, G. L. and Webster, A. D. B. (1980). Diagnosis and treatment of immunodeficiency diseases. p. 7. (Oxford: Blackwell)
5. Kyong, C. U., Virella, D., Fudenberg, H. W. and Darby, C. P. (1978). X-linked immunodeficiency with increased IgM: clinical, ethnic and immunologic heterogeneity. *Pediatr. Res.*, **12**, 1024–6
6. Webster, A. D. B. (1984). Echovirus disease in hypogammaglobulinaemia patients. *Clin. Rheumatic Dis.*, **10**, 189–203
7. Bernatowska, E. and Madalinski, K. (1987). Intravenous immunoglobulin therapy in progressive encephalitis in X-linked hypogammaglobulinaemia. *Acta Pediatr. Scand.*, **76**, 155–3
8. Erlendsson, K., Swartz, T. and Dwyer, J. M. (1985). Successful reversal of echovirus encephalitis in X-linked hypogammaglobulinaemia by intraventricular administration of immunoglobulin. *N. Engl. J. Med.*, **312**, 351–3
9. Roifman, C. M., Rao, C. P., Lederman, H. M., Lavi, S., Quinn, P. and Gelfand, E. W. (1986). Increased susceptibility to Mycoplasma infection in patients with hypogammaglobulinaemia. *Am. J. Med.*, **80**, 590–4
10. Taylor-Robinson, D. and McCormack, W. M. (1980). The genital mycoplasmas. *N. Engl. J. Med.*, **302**, 1003–10 and 1063–7
11. Webster, A. D. B., Furr, P. M., Hughes-Jones, N. C., Gorick, B. D. and Taylor-Robinson, D. (1988). Critical dependence on antibody for defence against mycoplasmas. *Clin. Exp. Immunol.* (In Press)
12. Taylor-Robinson, D., Furr P. M. and Webster, A. D. B. (1985). Ureaplasma urealyticum causing persistent urethritis in a patient with hypogammaglobulinaemia. *Genitourin. Med.*, **61**, 404–8
13. The European Group for Immunodeficiencies (EGID) (1986). Intravenous gammaglobulin for immunodeficiency: report. *Clin. Exp. Immunol.*, **65**, 683–90
14 Prince, A. M., Piet, M. J. P. and Horowitz, B. (1986). Effect of Cohn fractionation conditions on infectivity of the AIDS virus. *N. Engl. J. Med.*, **314**, 386–7
15 Roifman, C. M., Levison, H. and Gelfand, E. W. (1987). High dose versus low dose intravenous immunoglobulin in hypogammaglobulinaemia and chronic lung disease. *Lancet*, **1**, 1075–7
16 Frøland, S. S. and Natvig, J. B. (1972). Surface-bound immunoglobulin on lymphocytes from normal and immunodeficient humans. *Scand. J. Immunol.*, **1**, 1
17. Golay, J. T. and Webster, A. D. B. (1986). B cells in patients with X-linked and 'common variable' hypogammaglobulinaemia. *Clin. Exp. Immunol.*, **65**, 100–4
18. Fu, S. M., Hurley, J. N., McCune, J. M., Kunkel, H. G. and Good, R. A. (1980). Pre-B cells and other possible precursor lymphoid cell lines derived from patients with X-linked agammaglobulinaemia. *J. Exp. Med.*, **152**, 1519
19. Conley, M. E., Brown, P., Pickard, A. R., Buckley, R. N., Miller, D. S., Raskind, W. H.,

Singer, J. W. and Fialkow, P. J. (1986). Expression of the gene defect in X-linked agammaglobulinaemia. *N. Engl. J. Med.*, **315**, 564-7

20. Fearon, E. R., Winkelstein, J. A., Civin, C. I., Pardoll, D. M. and Vogelstein, B. (1987). Carrier detection in X-linked agammaglobulinaemia by analysis of X-chromosome inactivation. *N. Engl. J. Med.*, **316**, 427

21. Matamoros, N., Abad, E. and Webster, A. D. B. (1982). LDH isoenzymes in the T lymphocytes of patients with primary hypogammaglobulinaemia. *Clin. Exp. Immunol.*, **50**, 617

22. Johnson, S. M., North, M. E., Asherson, G. L., Allsop, J., Watts, R. W. E. and Webster, A. D. B. (1977). Lymphocyte purine 5'nucleotidase deficiency in primary hypogammaglobulinaemia. *Lancet*, **1**, 168

23. Seigal, F. R., Seigal, M. and Good, R. A. (1976). Suppression of B-cell differentiation by leucocytes from hypogammaglobulinaemic patients. *J. Clin. Invest.*, **58**, 109

24. Rozynska, K. E., Spickett, G., Bryant, A., Webster, A. D. B. and Farrant, J. (1988). Cellular defects in immunodeficiency: a comparison between acquired hypogammaglobulinaemia and X-linked agammaglobulinaemia. In press

25. Kwan, S-P., Kunkel, L., Bruns, G., Wedgwood, R. J., Latt, S. and Rosen, F. S. (1986). Mapping of the X-linked agammaglobulinaemia locus by use of restriction fragment-length polymorphisms. *J. Clin. Invest.*, **77**, 649-52

26. Mensink, E. J. B. M., Thompson, A., Schot, J. D. L., Kraakman, M. E. M., Sandkuyl, L. and Schuurman, R. K. B. (1987). Genetic heterogeneity in X-linked agammaglobulinaemia complicates carrier detection and prenatal diagnosis. *Clin. Genet.* **31**, 91-6

27. Malcolm, S., de Saint Basile, G., Arveiler, B., Lau, Y. L., Fischer, A., Griscelli, C., Debre, M., Mandel, J. L., Callard, R. E., Robertson, M. E., Goodship, J. A., Pembrey, M. E. and Levinsky, R. J. (1987). Close linkage of random DNA fragments from Xq21.3-22 to X-linked agammaglobulinaemia (XLA) *Hum. Genet.*, **77**, 172-4

28. Linch, D. C. and Levinsky, R. J. (1983). Prenatal diagnosis of foetal immunological disorders, *Br. Med. Bull.*, **39**, 399-404

29. Purtilo, D. T., Cassel C. K., Young, J. P., Harper, R., Stephenson, S. R., Landing, B. H. and Jawter, G. F. (1975). X-linked recessive progressive combined variable immunodeficiency (Duncan's disease). *Lancet*, **1**, 935-40

30. Sakamoto, K., Freed, H. J. and Purtilo, D. T. (1980). Antibody responses to Epstein-Barr virus in families with the X-linked lymphoproliferative syndrome. *J. Immunol.*, **125**, 921-5

31. Hanto, D. W., Frizzera, G., Gajl-Pecjalska, K. J. and Simmonds, R. C. (1985). Epstein-Barr virus, immunodeficiency and B cell lymphoproliferation. *Transplantation*, **39**, 461-72

32. Harada, S., Bechtold, T., Seeley, J. K. and Purtilo, D. T. (1982). Cell-mediated immunity to Epstein-Barr virus (EBV) and natural killer (NK)-cell activity in the X-linked lymphoproliferative syndrome. *Int. J. Cancer*, **30**, 739

33. Skare, J. C., Milunsky, A., Byron, K. S. and Sullivan, J. L. (1987). Mapping the X-linked lymphoproliferative syndrome. *Proc. Natl. Acad. Sci.*, **84**, 2015-18

34. Kinlen, L. J., Webster, A. D. B., Bird, A. G., Haile, R., Peto, J., Soothill, J. F. and Thompson, R. A. (1985). Prospective study of cancer in patients with hypogammaglobulinaemia. *Lancet*, **1**, 263-6

35. Webster, A. D. B., Platts-Mills, T. A. E., Jannossy, G., Morgan, M. and Asherson, G. L. (1981). Autoimmune blood dyscrasias in five patients with hypogammaglobulinaemia: response of neutropenia to Vincristine. *J. Clin. Immunol.*, **1**, 113-18

36. Friedman, J. M., Fialkow, P. J., Davis, S. D., Ochs, H. D. and Wedgwood, R. J. (1977). Autoimmunity in the relatives of patients with immunodeficiency diseases. *Clin. Exp. Immunol.*, **28**, 375

37. Kushner, D. S., Dubin, A., Donlon, W. P. and Bronsky, D. (1960). Familial hypogammaglobulinaemia, splenomegaly and leukopenia. *Am. J. Med.*, **29**, 33

38. Webster, A. D. B. and Asherson, G. L. (1974). Identification and function of T cells in the peripheral blood of patients with hypogammaglobulinaemia. *Clin. Exp. Immunol.*, **18**, 499

39. Waldmann, T. A., Durm, M., Broder, S., Blackman, M., Blaese, R. M. and Strober, W. (1974). Role of suppressor cells in pathogenesis of common variable hypogammaglobulinaemia. *Lancet*, **2**, 609

40. Platts-Mills, T. A. E., DeGast, G. C., Webster, A. D. B., Asherson, G. L. and Wilkins, S. R. (1981). Two immunologically distinct forms of late-onset hypogammaglobulinaemia. *Clin.*

Exp. Immunol., **44**, 383–8
41. Ziegler-Heitbrock, H. W. L., Schramm, W., Stachel, P., Rumpold, H., Kraft, D., Wermcke, D., Von Der Helm, K., Eberle, J., Deinhardt, F., Rieber, E. P. and Riethmüller, G. (1985). Expansion of a minor subpopulation of peripheral blood lymphocytes (T8/Leu7⁺) in patients with haemophilia. *Clin. Exp. Immunol.*, **61**, 633–41
42. De Gast, G., Wilkins, S. R., Webster, A. D. B., Rickinson, A. and Platts-Mills, T. A. E. (1980). Functional 'immaturity' of isolated B cells from patients with hypoglobulinaemia. *Clin. Exp. Immunol.*, **42**, 535
43. Brenner, M. K., North, M. E., Chadda, H. R., Newton, C. A., Malkovsky, K., Webster, A. D. B. and Farrant, J. (1984). The role of B cell differentiation factors and specific T cell help in the pathogenesis of primary hypogammaglobulinaemia. *Eur. J. Immunol.*, **14**, 1021–7
44. Shah, T., Webster, A. D. B. and Peters, T. J. (1983). Lymphocyte enzyme activities in immunodeficiency syndromes with particular reference to common variable hypogammaglobulinaemia. *Clin. Exp. Immunol.*, **53**, 413–22
45. Thompson, L. F., Saxon, A., O'Connor, R. D. and Fox, R. I. (1983). Ecto-5'-nucleotidase activity in human T cell subsets. *J. Clin. Invest.*, **71**, 892–4
46. Webster, A. D. B. (1978). Lymphocyte ecto 5'-nucleotidase deficiency. CIBA Foundation Symposium 68 (new series) p. 135. (Amsterdam: Excerpta Medica)
47. Shah, T., Farrant, J., Webster, A. D. B. and Peters, T. J. (1988). *In vivo* and *in vitro* immunoglobulin production after inhibition of lymphocyte ecto 5'-nucleotidase (submitted)
48. Shah, T., Webster, A. D. B. and Peters, T. J. (1984). Kinetic properties of 5'-nucleotidase in blood lymphocytes from healthy subjects, immunodeficient patients and cord blood. *Clin. Exp. Immunol.*, **57**, 149–54
49. Mannhalter, J. W., Zlabinger, G. J. and Eibl, M. M. (1984). Defective macrophage-T cell interaction in common varied immunodeficiency. *Prog. Immunodeficiency Res. Ther.*, **1**, 147 (Elsevier)
50. Luquetti, A., Newton, C. A. and Webster, A. D. B. (1981). Cellular immunity in primary hypogammaglobulinaemia: evidence for a generalised lymphocyte defect in some patients with 'common' variable hypogammaglobulinaemia. *Allergol. et Immunopathol.*, **9**, 295–306
51. Preud'Homme, J. L., Griscelli, C. and Seligmann, M. (1973). Immunoglobulins on the surface of lymphocytes in 50 patients with primary immunodeficiency diseases. *Clin. Immunol. Immunopath.*, **1**, 241
52. Pereira, F. S., Webster, A. D. B. and Platts-Mills, T. A. E. (1982). Immature B cells in fetal development and immunodeficiency. Studies of IgM, IgG, IgA and IgD production *in vitro* using Epstein–Barr virus activation. *Eur. J. Immunol.*, **12**, 540–6
53. Jeunet, F. J. and Good, R. A. (1968). Thymoma, immunologic deficiencies and hematological abnormalities. In Gergsma D. (ed.) *Immunologic Deficiency Diseases in Man.* (New York: The National Foundation, March of Dimes)
54. Hayward, A. R., Paolucci, P., Webster, A. D. B. and Kohler, P. (1982). Pre-B cell suppression by thymoma patient lymphocytes. *Clin. Exp. Immunol.*, **48**, 437–42
55. Brenner, M. K., Reittie, J. G. C., Chadda, H. R., Pollock, A. and Asherson, G. L. (1984). Thymoma and hypogammaglobulinaemia with and without T-suppressor cells. *Clin. Exp. Immunol.*, **58**, 619–24
56. Ho, M. (1984). Immunology of cytomegalovirus: immunosuppressive effects during infection. *Birth defects*, **20**, 131–47
57. Carney, W. P., Rubin, R. H., Hoffman, R. A., Hansen, W. P., Healey, K. and Hirsh, M. S. (1981). Analysis of T lymphocyte subsets in cytomegaloviral mononucleosis. *J. Immunol.*, **126**, 2114–16
58. Gehrz, R. C., Christianson, W. R., Linner, K. M., Conroy, M. M., McCue, S. A. and Balfour, H. H. (1981). Cytomegalovirus – specific humoral and cellular immune responses in human pregnancy. *J. Infect. Dis.*, **143**, 391–5
59. Lane, H. C., Masur, H., Edgar, L. C., Whales, G., Rook, A. H. and Fauci, A. S. (1983). Abnormalities of B-cell activation and immunoregulation in patients with the acquired immunodeficiency syndrome. *N. Engl. J. Med.*, **309**, 453
60. Schnittman, S. M., Lane, H. C., Higgins, S. E., Folks, T. and Fauci, A. S. (1986). Direct polyclonal activation of human B lymphocytes by the acquired immune deficiency syndrome virus. *Science*, **233**, 1084–6
61. Pahwa, R., Good, R. A. and Pahwa, S. (1987). Prematurity, hypogammaglobulinaemia

and neuropathology with human immunodeficiency virus (HIV) infection. *Proc. Natl. Acad. Sci. USA*, **84**, 3827-30

62. Webster, A. D. B., Malkovsky, M., Patterson, S., North, M., Dalgleish, A. G., Beattie, R., Asherson, G. L. and Weiss, R. A. (1986). Isolation of retroviruses from two patients with 'common variable' hypogammaglobulinaemia. *Lancet*, **1**, 581-3

63. Spickett, G. P., Millrain, M., North, M., Griffiths, J., Patterson, S. and Webster, A. D. B. (1988). Role of retroviruses in acquired hypogammaglobulinaemia. *Clin. Exp. Immunol.*, submitted

64. Gendelman, H. E., Narayan, O., Molineaux, S., Clements, J. E. and Ghotbi, Z. (1985). Slow, persistent replication of lentiviruses: role of tissue macrophages and macrophage precursors in bone marrow. *Proc. Natl. Acad. Sci. USA*, **82**, 7086-90

65. Chapel, H. M. and Bunch, C. (1988). Mechanisms of infection in chronic lymphocytic leukaemia. *Sem. Haematol.*, **24**, 291-6

66. Carter, A., Silvian, I., Tatoroky, I. and Spira, G. (1986). Impaired immunoglobulin synthesis in multiple myeloma: a B-cell dysfunction. *Am. J. Hematol.*, **22**, 143-54

3
Immunoglobulin Replacement Therapy

C. CUNNINGHAM-RUNDLES

HISTORICAL DEVELOPMENT

The basic concept that specific plasma substances can be important in host defence is a central theme in the historical development of immunology. As early as 1890, von Behring and Kitasato discovered that neutralizing antisera to tetanus and diphtheria toxins could be produced in animals by prior exposure to antigen and that the active principle was found in plasma[1]. Soon after, Erhlich's reports described the biological activities of diphtheria antitoxins[2]. In time, reports of other antitoxins, bacteriolysins, precipitins and agglutinins were described, each of them found to be active plasma principals capable of transfer by plasma. As this field developed, the ability of neutrophils to phagocytose encapsulated bacteria was found to be dependent upon the exposure of the bacterial surfaces to serum[3]. Later, the need for type-specific antibodies directed to bacterial cell structures was clarified[4]. Other mechanisms of microbial destruction by serum factors were then elucidated – for example, the bacteriolysis of cholera vibrios and Gram negative organisms was shown to be dependent upon interactions between specific antibodies and bacterial cell wall structures[5]. Bordet then showed that the lysis of erythrocytes was accomplished by serum antibody and complement[6]. This led to studies of complement fixation and opened the door to a number of diagnostic possibilities which were first applied to the infectious diseases. All of the above developments were closely linked to the emerging fields of medical microbiology, haematology and immunology.

The term antibody, which first appeared in the reports of Ehrlich in connection with studies of plant toxins in 1891[7], was later used by other authors as a general term for soluble biological factors. Later it became clear that placental extracts and plasma itself could be treated in such a way as to concentrate the active elements[8,9]. McKhann and co-workers, for example, isolated globulins from placental extracts using ammonium sulphate, to produce an anti-measles serum[8] and later Cohn et al.[9] introduced cold ethanol

43

fractionation to produce 'immune globulin (human)' as these substances were first termed in 1936[10]. Immunoglobulin globulin (human)' was used in the prevention or modification of measles in 1935, and the alcohol fractionated material was first used for prophylaxis against measles and hepatitis A in 1945[8, 11, 12].

In 1952 immunoglobulin concentrates were first used in the treatment of human immunodeficiency disease, although the report of the first case refrains from equating 'antibody' with gammaglobulin, stating that 'to speak of gammaglobulin and antibody interchangeably is probably incorrect'[13]. However, it was assumed that anti-pneumococcal antibody was contained in the gammaglobulin fraction, since the first patient treated no longer had periodic pneumococcal sepsis. Additionally, immune antibodies to diphtheria and typhoid were believed to be present in the concentrates since immunity to these latter organisms was demonstrated in the serum of this patient after treatment, but not before.

Currently, intramuscular immunoglobulin is produced from pools of plasma derived from outdated blood obtained from 500–2000 volunteer or paid donors. In some areas placental blood is used instead. The plasma is treated with alcohol to precipitate the immunoglobulin-containing fraction and after further purification, the standard preparation is approximately 15% in immunoglobulin, of which 85% is IgG, 10% is IgM and 5% is IgA[14]. Other serum proteins are present in trace amounts.

Another mode of therapy for antibody replacement, that of plasma infusion, has also been used in the primary immunodeficiency diseases[15,16]. While higher levels of serum immunoglobulins can be achieved by this method of treatment, it is cumbersome, and must involve donors of known medical history who are screened for hepatitis, and more recently HIV. Another drawback to plasma infusion is that the donated immunoglobulin can only confer the antigenic experience of the donor, and a broad range of antibodies in high titre is not likely to be present.

Intravenous infusion of gammaglobulin concentrates were considered and tried in the 1950s and 1960s, but these infusions resulted in severe reactions in a number of instances. However, over time, various methods to modify the immunoglobulin solutions were devised to produce products suitable for intravenous use. The following methods have been found satisfactory:

(1) Enzymatic action on immunoglobulin[17, 18];

(2) Stabilization of immunoglobulin by exposure to acid with traces of pepsin[19];

(3) Addition of chemical groups to prevent aggregation[20];

(4) Reduction, sulphonation or reduction followed by alkylation[21, 22];

(5) Addition of stabilizers (maltose, sucrose, albumin)[22, 23];

(6) Filtration[23];

(7) Precipitation of aggregates by polyethylene glycol[24].

Table 3.1 Characteristics of intravenous immunoglobulin preparations[14]

Name of product	Manufacturer/ Distributor	Method of preparation	IgA (mg/ml)	IgM Content (mg/ml)	IgG1 Content in % of total IgG	IgG2	IgG3	IgG4	% split Products†
Rhôdiglobin	Merieux	plasmin[17]	0.14	0.05	18.5	80.0	0	1.5	65
Gamma-venin	Behring-Werke	pepsin[18]	>6.5	<0.05	n.t.	n.t.	n.t.	n.t.	86
Sandoglobulin	Sandoz	pH 4.0 treated[19]	0.72	0.11	60.5	30.2	6.6	2.6	6
Intraglobulin	Biotest	B-propiolactone[20]	0.12	<0.05	64.3	34.5	0	1.2	0
Venilon	Teijin Institute	sulphonation[21]	0.32	0.40	69.0	29.0	0	1.8	0
Gamimune	Cutter Laboratories*	reduction, alkylation maltose stabilized[22]	0.27	0.10	70.2	28.2	0	1.6	1
Gammonativ	KabiVitrum	absorption by DEAE Sephadex, albumin stabilized[23]	<0.10	<0.05	61.6	33.0	4.5	0.7	0
Endobulin	Immuno	treatment with PEG[24]	0.10	0.19	64.1	30.3	4.0	1.5	1
Gammagard	Hyland-Travenol	absorption by DEAE Sephadex[25]	–	–	–	–	–	–	–
Human gammaglobulin intramuscular	Many producers	cold alcohol fraction, no further treatment	1.16	0.19	74.7	20.8	2.7	1.8	0

Data from Romer[14]

*Cutter Laboratories new IVGG is not reduced or alkylated but is maltose stabilized and kept at pH 4.25

†% split products performed by Ultragel ACA 34 chromotography

n.t. = not tested

45

The characteristics of these preparations are given in Table 3.1. In the past 10 years, in particular, the development of intravenous immunoglobulins has provided a substantial therapeutic advance in the treatment of antibody deficiency because large doses of immunoglobulin, containing a great diversity of antibodies, can safely be given in a concentrated form. The best method of preparation is not established; in fact, any method which produces an immunoglobulin concentrate containing intact and unmodified immunoglobulin in a form suitable for intravenous administration is satisfactory. Since enzyme-treated or reduced and alkylated immunoglobulin has been shown to have reduced effector functions in terms of opsonic capacity[25, 26] or fixation of complement[27, 28], these treatments are not usually favoured[29]. There is also a general consensus that such concentrates should contain IgG subclasses in the approximate proportions present in normal plasma and that no preservatives be added[29].

SAFETY

The issue of safety is a complex one, because both the intramuscular injection or intravenous infusion of immunoglobulin concentrates has been, at times, associated with immediate or delayed adverse reactions; there is also the potential for transmitting various viruses, and the possibility of causing immunomodulation.

Injection and infusion reactions

Intramuscular injections of immunoglobulin can produce a spectrum of adverse effects which have been observed and reported since the first of these preparations were administered[30–33]. About 10% of intramuscular injections are associated with reactions, and in a large study one death occurred[31]. Most reactions are mild, and include aches, back pain or chills. More rarely, nausea, vomiting, flushing, chest pain or mild fever are reported. The most common complaint is local pain at the site of the injection which may last for several days[31–33].

Because of side-effects to the intramuscular injections and evidence that immunoglobulin given intramuscularly or subcutaneously was only slowly absorbed into the systemic circulation[34], attempts were made to infuse the standard intramuscular solutions intravenously, but the incidence of adverse effects was unacceptable. In 1962, Barandun and colleagues administered 110 ml of a 1.45% gammaglobulin solution intended for intramuscular injection into each of 70 individuals[35]. They found that of 55 subjects who were not antibody deficient, 12.7% had an adverse reaction, while 14 of 15 with antibody deficiency (93.3%) had an adverse reaction.

The adverse effects were either immediate, beginning within minutes of starting the infusion, or delayed, occurring 1–2 hours after the infusion was completed. The immediate reactions consisted of flushing of the face, a feeling of oppression in the chest, lumbar pain, tachycardia, tachypnoea and shortness of breath. The delayed reactions were similar although some were mild with only chills and a slight rise in temperature . Severe reactions were almost exclusively limited to the antibody deficiency group. Here the course was found to resemble anaphylaxis, including chills, dyspnoea, sense of oppression, nausea, vomiting, lumbar pain, circulatory collapse, loss of consciousness and high fever. Such reactions, even those which were very severe, usually subsided in 3–4 hours. After having a reaction patients were refractory to subsequent reactions for about 5 days.

The reason for these reactions is generally believed to be due to complement activation by aggregates in the gammaglobulin[30, 33, 35]. However, this explanation is certainly not a complete one since it does not explain why hypogammaglobulinaemic patients are so much more likely to react than individuals with normal antibody levels; unless one assumes that hypogammaglobulinaemic patients have a reduced ability to clear immune complexes from the blood and are therefore more likely to experience complement activation. While this might be true, it has not been demonstrated.

Barandun and colleagues showed that ultracentrifuged immunoglobulin concentrates also produced reactions in antibody deficient patients. Because of this, they proposed that the retention of microbial antigens in the blood of hypogammaglobulinaemic patients could form antigen-antibody complexes with the infused antibody[35]. These complexes could activate the complement system. In support of this, they found that pepsin-treated, or pH 4.0 treated immunoglobulin had lost anti-complementary activity and could be infused without ill effects[35].

Despite evidence that the infusion of immunoglobulin aggregates can activate complement and result in adverse effects[35], there are obviously still many unresolved questions. Modest complement activation may often accompany the intravenous infusion of immunoglobulin, but this is not associated with clinical reactions[36]. In addition, we have found that circulating immune complexes are commonly present post-infusion – again, having no relationship to adverse effects[36, 37]. One antigen we have identified in such complexes is bovine casein, a dietary antigen absorbed from the intestinal tract in hypogammaglobulinaemic individuals[37].

There are additional possible causes of reactions, for example kallikreins[38], or other contaminants of blood processing. Some of these factors could lead to the leukopenia which is sometimes observed post-infusion[39]. Prostaglandin-like materials have also been implicated, since aspirin has been reported to alleviate some reactions[40]. IgE in the infused immunoglobulin is another possible cause of reactions since serum IgE levels are found to increase post-infusion, and IgE may be present in these concentrates[41].

Another unresolved question has been the nature of the refractory period which occurs after a reaction has occurred[35]. One assumes that some mediator has been depleted and cannot be restored for 4–5 days, but the nature of this substance is not known.

Antibodies to IgA

Autologous antibodies to IgA were first recognized in human sera in 1968[42]. These antibodies are present in up to 40% of sera of IgA deficient donors[43],

Table 3.2 Cases of hepatitis traceable to immunoglobulins

Patients	Location date	Dose	Product	Producer	Source of plasma	Patients with Abnormal LFT's/ total treated	Abnormal LFT's noted	Outcome	Comment	Reference
Normals	India, 1979	i.m. dose	intramuscular immunoglobulin	Commercial laboratory	India	?/325	78–172 days after injection	38% had jaundice	HBsAg+	52
Unknown	USA	i.m. dose	intramuscular immunoglobulin	not stated	USA	unknown	unknown	unknown	Made from plasma not screened for HbsAG	51
Hypogammaglobulinaemia, XLA	London, 1983	$200\,mg\,kg^{-1}$ (2 weeks)$^{-1}$, i.v.	intravenous immunoglobulin	British Blood Products Laboratory	UK	12/12	1–3 months after infusion	1 patient developed marrow hypoplasia	3 had liver biopsies, confirmed hepatitis	53
Hypogammaglobulinaemia	Seattle, 1983	$400\,mg\,kg^{-1}$ (4 weeks)$^{-1}$, i.v.	intravenous immunoglobulin	Hyland	USA	9/16	noted 2 years after study started	1 patient oedema, ascites, jaundice		54

Hypogammaglobulinaemia	Sweden, USA, 1984-1985	$75\,mg\,kg^{-1}$ or $300\,mg\,kg^{-1}$ i.v. (3 weeks)$^{-1}$	intravenous immunoglobulin	Kabi-Vitrum	Sweden, USA	6/22	1-3 months after infusion	1 patient died coronary, 'grossly cirrhotic' liver found		55
IgG subclass deficient	Sweden, USA, 1984-1985	$50\,mg\,kg^{-1}$ i.v. (4 weeks)$^{-1}$	intravenous immunoglobulin	Kabi-Vitrum	Sweden, USA	3/22	1-2 years after infusion	I died, uncertain cause, with oedema	3 had liver biopsies, chronic active hepatitis	55
Normal subjects	Sweden, 1985	2.5 g	intravenous immunoglobulin	Kabi-Vitrum	Sweden	2/?	6-7 months after infusion	chronic persistent hepatitis (1), chronic active hepatitis (1)	biopsy showed chronic active hepatitis, chronic persistent (1), chronic active (1) hepatitis	56
Hypogammaglobulinaemia	Sweden, 1985	5-15 g	intravenous immunoglobulin	Kabi-Vitrum	Sweden	2/? 2/?	18 months after infusion		biopsy showed chronic active hepatitis	56

and in 20% of patients with common varied immunodeficiency[44]. Infusion of blood or blood products containing IgA into a recipient who has circulating anti-IgA antibodies can result in severe infusion reactions; for this reason, an occasional hypogammaglobulinaemic individual has experienced adverse reactions after injection or infusion of immunoglobulin since these concentrates contain sufficient IgA to react with circulating anti-IgA antibody.

Such reactions (especially after intraveneous immunoglobulin) can be extremely severe, and dramatic complement activation has been demonstrated as well as long-term persistence of C3A in the serum[45]. Anti-IgA antibodies are usually of the IgG isotype, but IgE anti-IgA antibody has also been identified[46].

Several immunoglobulin products intended for intravenous infusion are depleted of IgA in the course of manufacturing. These have been successfully used for hypogammaglobulinaemic patients who require antibody treatment and have known anti-IgA antibodies[47,48]. Since immunoglobulin is now also recommended for the 12–18% of IgA deficient individuals who are also IgG2 subclass deficient and have recurrent infections, an IgA-depleted immunoglobulin might be a good choice for these patients also[49].

Transmission of virus

A major worry about the infusion of blood and blood products is the potential for the transmission of virus. A 1982 review of the incidence of hepatitis after the infusion of plasma derivatives drew attention to the high risk of non-A non-B hepatitis after receiving factor VIII and factor IX concentrates[50]. In contrast, human immunoglobulin concentrates for intravenous injection have not been noted for the transmission of hepatitis, although there are a few cases of hepatitis on record which are traceable to injections of intramuscular immunoglobulins (Table 3.2)[51,52].

However, several instances of hepatitis outbreaks have already been reported involving hypogammaglobulinaemic patients who have received intravenous immunoglobulins[53-56]. Since in each case the starting immunoglobulin solution was the same as for intramuscular use, it is mysterious why some intravenous preparations are infective. While these observations have induced caution about the use of intravenous preparations, in most of the instances reported, selected batches or lots of immunoglobulin have been implicated. More importantly, large numbers of infusions of intravenous immunoglobulin have been given to numerous patients without any alteration of liver enzymes over long periods of close observation.

Also of concern has been the possibility that immunoglobulin concentrates could transmit HIVS. Various experiments suggest that immunoglobulin concentrates cannot transmit these viruses[57]. This has been determined by purposeful contamination of plasma with the virus, and then subsequent testing of residual infectivity at various points along the preparative cycle[58]. It appears that several steps in the scheme remove this virus. At this time there are no known cases of AIDS due to the use of immunoglobulin concentrates. However, passive infusion of antibody to the virus can render the recipient antibody positive for up to 6 months[59].

Immunomodulation

In addition to the intentional effect of restoring humoral immunity, the infusion of immunoglobulin could exert separate immunomodulating effects. Durandy *et al.* described an immunosuppressive effect of intramuscular immunoglobulin given to children with recurrent infections who were not hypogammaglobulinaemic, and in some hypogammaglobulinaemic patients who received a plasmin-treated intravenous immunoglobulin[60]. In other studies, the addition of post-infusion serum of hypogammaglobulinaemic patients to pokeweed-stimulated cultures of mononuclear cells of normal donors suppressed immunoglobulin synthesis in these cultures (as compared to additions of pre-infusion samples of serum)[61,62,63].

In other studies of patients with ITP, large doses of intravenous immunoglobulin have been shown to produce a temporary blockade of Fc receptors on cells of the reticuloendothelial system[64,65]. Peripheral monocyte Fc receptors are reduced in number following treatment with intravenous immunoglobulin[66] and natural killer cell activity is temporarily diminished[67]. Some investigators have proposed possible anti-idiotypic interactions[68]. In most of the above instances, the binding of the Fc portion of the administered immunoglobulin with cell-bound Fc receptors is essential for the modulating effect. At present, these effects are of academic interest only and no significant or lasting suppressive effects have been documented in immunodeficient patients receiving immunoglobulin.

EFFICACY

That gammaglobulin treatment is efficacious for patients with humoral immunodeficiency was quickly apparent to not only the first investigator who used immunoglobulin concentrates, but to all subsequent physicians caring for these patients[31-33]. What has been harder to decide is the maximally effective and practical dose of intramuscular immunoglobulin, and for intravenous immunoglobulins, both the proper dose and the product type. The issue is further complicated because universal guidelines cannot be applied to individual patients because their requirements differ.

Intramuscular immunoglobulin

The first immunodeficient patient treated with 'immunoglobulin (human)' was 8 years old and received 3.2 g of gammaglobulin subcutaneously at intervals of 1 month[13]. This dose was found to increase the amount of gammaglobulin observed on serum electrophoresis; the interval was chosen because of a gradual decline in the serum level over a 4-week period. The original dose was chosen by estimate, but it is similar to the dose of $100 \, \text{mg} \, \text{kg}^{-1} \, \text{month}^{-1}$ which has since been generally recommended. This dose can satisfactorily raise the serum IgG level from near zero to 100 or 150 mg/dl, a level which is considered to be the minimum level necessary to prevent infections[32].

A suitable interval between doses was later established in studies of other patients in whom the half-life of immunoglobulin was found to range between 15 and 30 days[69]. However, since the half-life of individual antibodies varies between 17 and 58 days[70], and the catabolism of IgG in hypogammaglobulinaemic patients is often delayed[71], it is difficult to offer any firm guidelines on dosage.

The recommended dose of $100\,mg\,kg^{-1}\,month^{-1}$ (or $25\,mg\,kg^{-1}\,week^{-1}$) made a clear impact on the incidence of morbidity (and mortality) in hypogammaglobulinaemic patients. In order to determine whether this dose was optimal, the Medical Research Council in Great Britain performed a trial in which patients treated with the usual dose of $25\,mg\,kg^{-1}\,week^{-1}$ were compared with patients receiving $50\,mg\,kg^{-1}\,week^{-1}$. The results showed that patients receiving the higher dose had significantly fewer infections[31]. However, the latter dose was not practical to administer since it would mean, for example, that 20 ml of a 15% solution (the usual concentration) would have to be administered weekly to a 60 kg patient. Thus the generally recommended dose for hypogammaglobulinaemic patients is based more upon expediency than the available clinical data.

Intravenous immunoglobulin

The use of intramuscular immunoglobulin changed the course of the humoral immunodeficiency diseases, but it is clear from the above discussion that the dose which could be given by the intramuscular route was not necessarily the optimally effective dose. In addition, patients with poor musculature could not be given adequate doses. Merely the pain of the injection (even at the recommended dose) could deter the patient (and the physician) from persisting. Attempts were made to give immunoglobulin concentrates intended for intramuscular injection by intravenous infusion. However, as discussed above, serious reactions occurred, particularly in immunodeficient individuals, and these efforts were soon abandoned. Various efforts to produce suitable intravenous immunoglobulins resulted in a group of products which could be safely infused.

As for the question of efficacy for these intravenous concentrates, the first proving ground was to establish that the intravenous forms were at least equally able to prevent infection in patients with humoral immunodeficiency when compared to intramuscular treatment. Several such studies have been performed, but the question of efficacy is entangled in the issues of choice of intravenous preparation, and doses used. One report of a cross-over trial in 34 patients compared the standard intramuscular dose of $100\,mg\,kg^{-1}\,month^{-1}$ with the same dose of a reduced and alkylated preparation given intravenously. Somewhat disconcertingly, the results showed that the intravenous immunoglobulin was associated with a higher incidence of infections (Table 3.3)[40]. While this may have been due to reporting artifacts stemming from the increased number of visits to the major medical centres made by the intravenously-infused patients, it still did not appear that intravenous treatment with the product used, at the dose given, was clearly preferable.

Table 3.3 Comparison of intramuscular and intravenous immunoglobulin and incidence of infection[40]

	Intravenous immunoglobulin*	Intramuscular immunoglobulin†
Number of patients	34	34
Percentage of patients with acute infections:		
Upper respiratory tract	85.3	50.0
Gastrointestinal tract	55.9	38.2
Otitis media	52.9	47.1
Bronchitis	50.0	41.2
Sinusitis	20.6	17.6
Oral	17.6	8.8
Conjunctival	29.4	26.5
Skin	29.4	32.4

*dose $100\,mg\,kg^{-1}\,month^{-1}$, reduced and alkylated immunoglobulin
†dose $100\,mg\,kg^{-1}\,month^{-1}$, standard solution

In another trial, a significant reduction in rate of infection was demonstrated for hypogammaglobulinaemic patients receiving 150 mg/kg intravenously (Table 3.4)[72]. Since the patients in both studies had been treated with the reduced and alkylated immunoglobulin, it seems plausible that a dose of 150 mg/kg of this product may be the minimum dose at which efficacy over intramuscular immunoglobulin can be shown.

Table 3.4 Trial to investigate rate of infection after intravenous or intramuscular treatment[72]

	Intravenous treatment*	Intramuscular treatment†
Number of patients	13	13
Number of acute infections	15	57
Acute infections/months therapy	0.067	0.295

*Dose, $150\,mg\,kg^{-1}\,month^{-1}$ reduced and alkylated immunoglobulin
†Dose, $100\,mg\,kg^{-1}\,month^{-1}$ standard solution

Other investigators have analysed the effects of intravenous immunoglobulin given at higher doses. We studied the dose of 300 mg/kg of a chemically intact immunoglobulin given at 3-week intervals as compared to prior therapy with intramuscular immunoglobulin at standard dosage. A highly significant overall improvement was observed (Table 3.5). While not all patients enrolled in this study improved, and subsequently several were treated with even higher doses, we concluded that $300\,mg\,kg^{-1}\,(3\,weeks)^{-1}$ of this immunoglobulin is a dose which benefits most patients[73].

Table 3.5 Effect of higher doses on intravenous or intramuscular treatment[73]

	Intravenous treatment*	Intramuscular treatment†
Number of patients	18	18
Days sick	258	834
Days on antibiotics	1820	3249

*Dose $300\,mg\,kg^{-1}(3\ weeks)^{-1}$. Chemically intact, pH 4.0 treated
†Dose 40–$80\,mg\,kg^{-1}$ (2 weeks)$^{-1}$, standard solution

In other studies, still higher doses of intravenous immunoglobulin have been tried. Monthly doses of $400\,mg/kg^{74}$, $500\,mg/kg$ over varied intervals determined by serum IgG levels[75], and $600\,mg/kg^{-1}$ month^{-1} [76] have been infused without ill effect, and sometimes with apparent benefit. It seems that overall, post-infusion serum IgG levels rise by approximately $250\,mg/dl$ for each $100\,mg$ of immunoglobulin/kg infused. However, individual patients can display marked differences in their apparent catabolic rate and some investigators have sought to individualize doses in order to establish a minimum trough value[77, 78].

Patients adequately treated with immunoglobulin concentrates show a significant improvement which is most obvious in the reduced frequency of respiratory tract infections, episodes of otitis, sinusititis and conjuctivitis. Patients who have more severe tissue damage, particularly severe pulmonary disease, do not show as much benefit, but some investigators use high doses of intravenous immunoglobulin in such patients with apparent benefit[76].

Another less responsive area is the gastrointestinal tract; patients who have chronic diarrhoea are not likely to improve [40, 72, 73]. In contrast, patients with joint pains and even objective joint swelling prior to intravenous therapy can experience dramatic improvement.

FUTURE DEVELOPMENTS

Home care, subcutaneous immunoglobulin infusion

As immunoglobulin usage expands and the emphasis upon patient independence increases, two newer aspects of immunoglobulin therapy are becoming important. Numerous investigators have found that hypogamma-globulinaemic patients can be satisfactorily enrolled in various home care programmes, in which either the patient or a registered nurse mixes intravenous immunoglobulin and starts the infusion. Most patients rely upon a pump to regulate the immunoglobulin flow; this method has been quite satisfactory for many patients. The costs are high, but are probably less than receiving treatment in a hospital setting; there is also less disruption of the patient's work or schooling.

Another advance is the use of subcutaneous immunoglobulin infusion which relies upon the slow subcutaneous infiltration of immunoglobulin concentrates by a pump mechanism which is loaded and operated by the patient[79, 80]. This method is inexpensive, because the immunoglobulin concentrates intended for intramuscular treatment are used, and it is capable of producing quite satisfactory levels of serum IgG. The disadvantage is that the patient must wear the pump for 3-4 hours several times a week to satisfactorily increase serum IgG levels.

Use in secondary immunodeficiency

Immunoglobulin replacement therapy is an unarguable necessity in the primary immune deficiency diseases. What is less clear are the potential benefits of immunoglobulin in situations of secondary antibody deficiency such as chronic lymphocytic leukaemia, after chemotherapy for cancer, nephrotic syndrome, fetal prematurity, protein loss, burns and bone marrow transplantation. In these situations, serum immunoglobulin levels may be significantly reduced, although antibody levels when investigated are more variably decreased. Some data have shown that intravenous immunoglobulin may be of benefit in patients with small cell carcinoma of the lung[81] and for patients who have sustained multiple trauma[82]. Sporadic reports comment upon the use of intravenous immunoglobulin in protein losing enteropathy[83], leukaemia[84] and burns[85]. Few large controlled studies have been done but at least four are now ongoing concerning the use of intravenous immuno-globulin in patients with chronic lymphocytic leukaemia, in fetal prematurity, in burns, and in bone marrow transplantation. Hopefully these studies will provide clear evidence for or against the premise that immunoglobulin replacement is useful in these situations.

Use in viral infections

High dose immunoglobulin therapy has been used in several studies for prophylaxis against infections with cytomegalovirus in bone marrow transplant recipients; some showed a positive effect[86, 87] while others had no effect[88]. Beneficial effects have also been shown for *Herpes zoster* infections in immunocompromised patients[89]. Intravenous immunoglobulin is also currently used in patients with AIDS but these studies have not been controlled and the results are difficult to assess[90, 91].

More recently, some patients diagnosed as having chronic Epstein-Barr virus infection have been treated with intravenous immunoglobulin, but since the syndrome is still very poorly defined, and the rationale for treatment is unclear, the available data remain anecdotal.

In one viral infection, the use of immunoglobulin replacement therapy appears to have an established role and to have produced results. This is for echovirus infections in patients with X-linked agammaglobulinaemia[92].

New products

Immunoglobulin therapy has recently expanded and regained interest, as a direct result of new methods of producing intravenous immunoglobulins which can be safely infused in large amounts. New areas being explored include the production of various hyperimmune globulins which could have a potential role in the prophylaxis of infectious disease. Manufacturers are also considering new methods to eliminate viruses from immunoglobulin and other plasma concentrates. A recent report appears promising[93].

References

1. Von Behring, E. and Kitasato, S. (1890). Ueber das Zustandekommen der Diptherie Immunitat und der Tetanus-Immunitat bei Thieren. *Dtsch. Med Wschr.*, **16**, 1113–15
2. Ehrlich, P. (1897). Die Wertbemessung des Diptherie-heilserums und deren theorestische grundlagen. *Klin. Jahrbuch*, **6**, 299–326
3. White, B. (1938). *The Biology of the Pneumococcus*. The Common Wealth Fund, New York. (This volume has been reprinted by the Harvard University Press, 1979)
4. Lancefield, R. C. (1928). The antigenic complex of *Streptococcus haemolyticus*. II. Chemical and immunologic properties of the protein fractions. *J. Exp. Med.*, **47**, 469–80
5. Taylor, P. W. (1983). Bactericidal and bacteriolytic activity of serum against Gram-negative bacteria. *Microbiol. Rev.*, **47**, 46–83
6. Bordet, J. (1909) *Studies on Immunology*. Translated by Gay, I. (New York: John Wiley)
7. Ehrich, P. (1957). *The Collected Papers of Paul Ehrlich*. Vol. 2. (New York: Pergamon)
8. McKhann, C. F. and Chu, F. T. (1933). Antibodies in placental extracts. *J. Infect. Dis.*, **52**, 266–77
9. Cohn, E. J., Strong, L. E., Hughes, W. L. *et al.* (1946). Preparation and properties of serum and plasma proteins. IV. A system for the separation into fractions of protein and lipoprotein components of biological tissues and fluids. *J. Am. Chem. Soc.*, **68**, 459–75
10. Eley, R. C., Green, A. A. and McKhann, C. F. (1936). The use of a blood coagulant extract from the human placenta in the treatment of hemophilia. *J. Pediatr.*, **8**, 135–47
11. McKhann, C. F., Green, A. A. and Coady, H. (1935). Factors influencing the effectiveness of placental extracts in the prevention and modification of measles. *J. Pediatr.*, **6**, 603–14
12. Stokes, J. and Neefe, J. R. (1945). Prevention and attenuation of infectious hepatitis by gammaglobulin; preliminary note. *J. Am. Med. Assoc*, **127**, 144–5
13. Bruton, O. C. (1952). Agammaglobulinemia. *Pediatrics*, **9**, 722–8
14. Romer, J. J., Morgenthaler, J. T., Scherz, R. and Skvaril, F. (1981). Characterization of various immunoglobulin preparations for intravenous application. *Vox Sang.*, **42**, 62–9
15. Stiehm, E. R., Vaerman, J. P. and Fudenberg, H. H. (1966). Plasma infusions in immunologic deficiency states: metabolic and therapeutic studies. *Blood*, **28**, 918–37
16. Buckley, R. H. (1972). Plasma therapy in immunodeficiency diseases. *Am. J. Dis. Child.*, **124**, 376–81
17. Sgouris, J. T. (1967). The preparation of plasmin-treated immune serum globulin for intravenous use. *Vox Sang.*, **13**, 571–84
18. Schultze, M. E. and Schwick, G. (1962). Uber neue Moglichkeiten Intravenoser Gammaglobulin-Applikation. *Dtsch. Med. Wschr.*, **87**, 1643–50
19. Barandun, S. (1964). Die Gammaglobulin-Therapic Chemische, immunologische und klinische. *Grundlagen. Bibl Haemat.*, **17**, 1–138
20. Stephan, W. (1969). Beseitigung der Komplement fixierung von γ-globulin durch chemische modifzierung mit B-Propiolacton. *Z. Klin. Chem. Biochem.*, **7**, 282–6
21. Ochs, H. D., Buckley, R. H., Pirofsky, B., Fischer, S. H., Rousell, R. H., Anderson, C. J. and Wedgwood, R. J. (1980). Safety and patient acceptability of intravenous immune globulin in 10% maltose. *Lancet*, **2**, 1158–9
22. Gronski, P., Hofstaetter, T., Kanzy, E. J., Luben, G. and Seiler, F. R. (1983). *S*-sulfonation: a reversible chemical modification of human immunoglobulins permitting intravenous application. I. Physicochemical and binding properties of *S*-sulfonated and reconstituted IgG. *Vox Sang.*, **45**, 144–54
23. Hanson, L. A., Bjorkander, J., Wadsworth, C. and Bake, B. (1982). Intravenous immuno-globulin in antibody deficiency syndromes (letter). *Lancet*, **1**, 396
24. Eibl, M. (1979). Intravenous immunoglobulins: clinical and experimental studies. In Alving, B. M. and Finlayson, J. S. (eds) *Immunoglobulins: Characteristics and Uses of Intravenous Preparations*. pp. 167–72. U.S. Department of Health and Human Services, DHHS Publication No. (FDA) 80-9005

25. Von Furth, R. and Leigh, P. C. J. (1981). Functional interactions of various commercial gammaglobulin preparations with *S. Aureus* and granulocytes. In *Immunohemotherapy, a Guide to Immunoglobulin Prophylaxis and Therapy*. pp. 181-90. (London: Academic Press)
26. Hetherington, S. V. and Giebnick, G. S. (1984). Opsonic activity of immunoglobulin prepared for intravenous use. *J. Lab. Clin. Med.*, **104**, 977-86
27. Cunningham-Rundles, C. (1984). Normalization of serum C1q after intravenous immunoglobulin infusion in hypogammaglobulinemia: dependence upon methods of immunoglobulin preparation. *Clin. Immunol. Immunopathol.*, **33**, 176-81
28. Bing, D. H. (1984). Complement interaction with immune serum globulin and immune globulin intravenous. *Am. J. Med.*, **76** (3A), 19-24
29. Appropriate uses of human immunoglobulin in clinical practice: memorandum of an IUIS/WHO meeting (1982). *Bull. World Health Organization*, **60**, 45-7
30. Gitlin, D. and Janeway, C. A. (1956). Agammaglobulinemia, congenital, acquired and transient forms. *Prog. Hematol.*, **1**, 318-29
31. Hill, L. E. (1971). Clinical features of hypogammaglobulinemia. *Medical Research Council Special Report Series*, **310**, 106
32. Janeway, C. A. and Rosen, F. S. (1966). The gamma globulins. IV. Therapeutic uses of gamma globulin. *N. Engl. J. Med.*, **275**, 826-31
33. Soothill, J. F. (1971). Reactions to immunoglobulin. *Medical Research Council Special Report Series*, **310**, 106
34. Smith, G. N., Griffiths, B., Mollison, D. and Mollison, P. L. (1972). Uptake of IgG after intramuscular and subcutaneous injection. *Lancet*, **1**, 1208-12
35. Barandun, S., Kistler, P., Jeunet, F. and Isliker, H. (1962). Intravenous administration of human γ-globulin. *Vox Sang.*, **7**, 157-74
36. Day, N. K., Good, R. A. and Wahn, V. (1986). Adverse reactions in selected patients following intravenous infusions of gammaglobulin. *Am. J. Med.*, **76**, 25-32
37. Cunningham-Rundles, C. and Carr, R. I. (1988). Dietary bovine antigens and immune complex formation after intravenous immune deficiency. *J. Clin. Immunol.*, **65**, 381-8
38. Alving, B. M., Tankersley, D. L., Mason, B. L., Rossi, F., Aronson, D. L. and Finlayson, J. S. (1979). Vasoactive enzymes in immunoglobulin preparations. In Alving, B. M. and Finlayson, J. S. (eds.) *Immunoglobulins: Characteristics and Uses of Intravenous Preparations*. pp. 167-72. U.S. Department of Health and Human Services, DHHS Publication No. (FDA) 80-9005
39. Eibl, M. M., Cairns, L. and Rosen, F. S. (1984). Safety and efficacy of a monomeric, functionally intact intravenous IgG preparation in patients with primary immunodeficiency syndromes. *Clin. Immunol. Immunopathol.*, **31**, 151-60
40. Ammann, A. J., Ashman, R. F., Buckley, R. H., Hardie, W. R., Krantmann, H. J., Nelson, J., Ochs, H., Stiehm, E. R., Tiller, T., Wara, D. W. and Wedgwood, R. (1982). Use of intravenous γ-globulin in antibody immunodeficiency: results of a multi center controlled trial. *Clin. Immunol. Immunopathol.*, **22**, 60-7
41. Newland, A. C., Macey, M. G. and Bubel, M. (1984). IgE in intravenous IgG (letter). *Lancet*, **1**, 1406
42. Vyas, G. N., Perkins, H. A. and Fudenberg, H. H. (1968). Anaphylactoid transfusion reactions associated with anti-IgA. *Lancet*, **2**, 3-12
43. Hammarstrom, L., Person, M. A. A. and Smith, C. I. E. (1983). Anti-IgA in selective IgA deficiency. *Scand. J. Immunol.*, **18**, 509
44. Wells, J. V., Buckley, R. H., Schanfield, M. S. and Fudenberg, H. H. (1971). Anaphylactic reactions to plasma infusions in patients with hypogammaglobulinemia and anti-IgA bodies. *Clin. Immunol. Immunopathol.*, **8**, 265-8
45. Good, R. A., Gupta, S., Pahwa, S. and Day, N. K. (1984). Evidence of persistent IgA/IgG circulating immune complexes associated with activation of the complement system in serum of a patient with common variable immune deficiency: anaphylactic reactions to intravenous gammaglobulin. *Acta Pathol. Microbiol. Immunol. Scand.* (Suppl.), **284**, 49-58
46. Burks, A. W., Sampson, H. A. and Buckley, R. H. (1986). Anaphylactic reactions after gammaglobulin administration in patients with hypogammaglobulinemia. *N. Engl. J. Med.*, **314**, 560-2
47. Hanson, L. A., Bjorkander, J., Ljunggren, J., Oxelius, V-A. and Wadsworth, C. (1979). In

Alving, B. M. and Finlayson, J. S. (eds.) *Immunoglobulin Characteristics and Uses of Intravenous Preparations.* pp. 150–4. US Department of Health and Human Services, DHHS. Publication No. (FDA) 80-9005

48. Cunningham-Rundles, C., Wong, S., Bjorkander, J. and Hanson, L. A. (1986). Use of an IgA-depleted intravenous immunoglobulin in a patient with an anti-IgA antibody. *Clin. Immunol. Immunopathol.*, **38**, 141–9

49. Bjorkander, J., Hammarstrom, L., Smith, C. I. E., Buckley, R. H., Cunningham-Rundles, C. and Hanson, L. A. (1988). Immunoglobulin prophylaxis in patients with antibody deficiency syndromes and anti-IgA antibodies (submitted)

50. Gerety, R. J. and Aronson, D. L. (1982). Plasma derivatives and viral hepatitis. *Transfusion*, **22**, 347–51

51. Tabor, E. and Gerety, R. (1979). Transmission of hepatitis B by immune serum globulin. *Lancet*, **2**, 1293

52. John, T. J., Ninan, G. T., Rajagopalan, M. S., John, F., Lewett, T. H., Francis, D. P. and Zuckerman, A. J. (1979). Epidemic hepatitis B caused by commercial human immunoglobulin. *Lancet*, **1**, 1074

53. Lever, A. M. L., Webster, A. D. B., Brown, D. and Thomas, H. C. (1984). Non-A non-B hepatitis occurring in agammaglobulinemic patients after intravenous immunoglobulin. *Lancet*, **2**, 1062–4

54. Ochs, H. D., Fischer, S. H., Virant, F. S., Lee, M. L., Kingdon, H. and Wedgwood, R. J. (1985). Non-A, non-B hepatitis and intravenous immunoglobulin. *Lancet*, **1**, 404–5

55. Bjorkander, J., Cunningham-Rundles, C., Lundin, P., Soderstrom, R., Olsson, R. and Hanson, L. A. (1988). Intravenous immunoglobulin prophylaxis in hypogammaglobulinemia causing liver damage. *Am. J. Med.*, **84**, 107–11

56. Weiland, O., Mattsson, L. and Glaumann, H. (1986). Non-A, non-B hepatitis after intravenous gammaglobulin (letter). *Lancet*, **1**, 976–7

57. CDC (1986). Safety of therapeutic immunoglobulin preparations with respect to transmission of human T-lymphotropic virus type III/lymphadenopathy associated virus infection. *Morbidity and Mortality Weekly Report*, **35**, 231–2

58. Wells, M. A., Wittele, A., Marcus-Sekura, C. *et al.* (1986). Chemical and physical inactivation (HTLV III) of human T-cell lymphotropic virus, Type III, during ethanol fractionation of plasma transfusion. *Transfusion*, **26**, 210–13

59. Tedder, R. S., Uttley, A. and Cheingsong-Popov, R. (1985). Safety of immunoglobulin preparation containing anti-HTLV-III (letter). *Lancet*, **1**, 815

60. Durandy, A., Fischer, A. and Griscelli, C. (1981). Dysfunction of pokeweed mitogen stimulated T and B responses induced by gammaglobulin treatment. *J. Clin. Invest.*, **67**, 867–77

61. Stohl, W. (1985). Modulation of the immune response by immunoglobulin for intravenous use. I. Inhibition of pokeweed mitogen-induced B cell differentiation. *Clin. Exp. Immunol.*, **62**, 200–7

62. Stohl, W., Cunningham-Rundles, C. and Mayer, L. F. (1986). Modulation of the immune response by immunoglobulin for intravenous use. II. Inhibitory effects of sera from treated patients. *Clin. Immunol. Immunopathol.*, **41**, 273–80

63. Bussel, J. B., Pahwa, S., Porges, A., Cunningham-Rundles, S., Koziner, B., Morell, A. and Barandun, S. (1986). Correlation of *in vitro* antibody synthesis with the outcome of intravenous gammaglobulin therapy in chronic ITP. *J. Clin. Immunol.*, **6**, 50–6

64. Fehr, J., Hoffmann, V. and Kapperler, U. (1982). Transient reversal of thrombocytopenia in idiopathic thrombocytopenic purpura by high-dose intravenous gammaglobulin. *N. Engl. J. Med.*, **306**, 745–50

65. Bussel, J. B., Kimberley, R. P., Inman, R. D., Schulman, I., Cunningham-Rundles, C., Smithwick, E. M., O'Malley, J., Barandun, S., Polk, J. R., Cheung, N. and Hilgartner, M. W. (1983). Use of intravenous gammaglobulin in patients with chronic ITP. *Blood*, **62**, 480–6

66. Kimberly, R. P., Salmon, J. E., Bussel, J. B., Crow, M. K. and Hilgartner, M. W. (1984). Modulation of mononuclear phagocyte function by intravenous gamma-globulin. *J. Immunol.*, **132**, 745–50

67. Engelhard, D., Waner, J. L., Kapoor, N. D. and Good, R. A. (1986). Effect of intravenous immune globulin on natural killer cell activity: possible association with autoimmune neutropenia and idiopathic thrombocytopenia. *J. Pediatr.*, **108** (1), 77–81

68. Sultan, Y., Kazatchkine, M. D., Maisonneuve, P. and Nydegger, U. E. (1984). Antiidiotypic suppression of autoantibodies to factor VIII (antihaemophilic factor) by highdose intravenous gammaglobulin. *Lancet*, **2**, 765-8
69. Dixon, F. J., Talmage, D. W., Maurer, P. H. and Deichmiller, M. (1952). The half life of homologous gammaglobulin (antibody) in several species. *J. Exp. Med.*, **96**, 313-16
70. Martin, C. M., Gordon, R. S. and McCullough, N. B. (1956). Acquired hypogammaglobulinemia in an adult. *N. Engl. J. Med.*, **254**, 449
71. Waldman, T. A. and Schwab, P. J. (1965). IgG (7S gammaglobulin) metabolism in hypogammaglobulinemia: studies in patients with defective gammaglobulin synthesis. *J. Clin Invest.*, **44**, 1523-33
72. Nolte, M. T., Pirofsky, B., Gerritz, G. A. and Goeding, B. (1979). Intravenous immunoglobulin therapy for antibody deficiency. *Clin. Exp, Immunol.*, **36**, 337
73. Cunningham-Rundles, C., Siegal, F. P., Smithwick, E. M., Cunningham-Rundles, S., Lion-Boule, A., O'Malley, J., Barandun, S. and Good, R. A. (1984). Efficacy of intravenous gammaglobulin in humoral immunodeficiency disease. *Ann. Intern. Med.*, **101**, 435-9
74. Ochs, H., Fisher, S. H., Wedgwood, R. J., Wara, D. W., Cowan, M. J., Amman, A. J., Saxon, A., Budinger, M. D., Allred, R. U. and Rousell, R. (1984). Comparison of high dose and low dose intravenous immunoglobulin therapy in patients with primary immunodeficiency disease. *Am. J. Med.*, **76** (3A), 78-81
75. Montanaro, A. and Pirofsky, B. (1984). Prolonged high dose intravenous immunoglobulin in patients with primary immunodeficiency states. *Am. J. Med.*, **76** (3A), 67-73
76. Roifman, C. M., Lederman, H. M., Lavis, S., Stein, L. D., Levinson, H. and Gelfand, E. W. (1985). Benefit of intravenous IgG replacement in hypogammaglobulinemic patients with chronic sinopulmonary disease. *Am. J. Med.*, **79**, 171-4
77. Schiff, R. I., Rudd, C., Johnson, R. and Buckley, R. H. (1984). Use of a new chemically modified intravenous IgG efficacy and attempts to individualize dosage. *Clin. Immunol. Immunopathol.*, **31**, 13-23
78. Schiff, R. I. (1985). Individualizing the dose of intravenous immune serum globulin for therapy of patients with primary humoral immunodeficiency. *Vox Sang.*, **49** Suppl. 1, 15-24
79. Vander Meer, J. W. M., Von Furth, R. and Roord, J. J. (1981). Subcutaneous administration of gammaglobulin. In Nydegger, U. E. (ed.) *Immunohemotherapy, a Guide to Immunoglobulin Prophylaxis and Therapy*. pp. 441-3. (London: Academic Press)
80. Berger, M., Cupps, T. R. and Fauci, A. S. (1980). Immunoglobulin replacement therapy by slow subcutaneous infusion. *Ann. Intern. Med.*, **93**, 55-6
81. Schmidt, R. E., Hartlapp, J. H., Niese, D., Illiger, H. J. and Stroehmann, I. (1984). Reduction of infection frequency by intravenous gammaglobulins during intensive induction therapy for small cell carcinoma of the lung. *Infection*, **12**, 167-70
82. Stamm, F. and Stoffel, D. (1985). Polyvalent immunoglobulins for prophylaxis of bacterial infections in patients following multiple trauma. A randomized, placebo-controlled study. *Intensive Care Med.*, **11**, 288-94
83. Giacomo, C. De, Maggiore, C., Scotta, M.S. and Ugazio, A. G. (1985). Administration of intravenous immunoglobulin in two children with hypogammaglobulinemia due to protein losing enteropathy. *Clin. Exp. Immunol.*, **60**, 447-8
84. Besa, E. C. (1984). Use of intravenous immunoglobulin in chronic lymphocytic leukemia. *Am. J. Med.*, **76**(3A), 209-18
85. Shirani, K. Z., Vaughan, G. M., McManus, A. T., Amy, B. W., McManus, W. F., Pruitt, B. A. Jr. and Mason, A. D. Jr. (1984). Replacement therapy with modified immunoglobulin G in burn patients: preliminary kinetic studies. *Am. J. Med.*, **76**(3A), 175-80
86. Condie, R. M. and O'Reilly, R. J. (1984). Prevention of cytomegalovirus infection by prophylaxis with an intravenous, hyperimmune, native, unmodified cytomegalovirus globulin. Randomized trial in bone marrow transplant recipients. *Am. J. Med.*, **76**(3A), 134-41
87. Winston, D. J., Ho, W. G., Lin, G. H., Budinger, M. D., Champlin, R. E. and Gale, R. P. (1984). Intravenous immunoglobulin for modification of cytomegalovirus infections associated with bone marrow transplantation: preliminary results of a controlled trial. *Am. J. Med.*, **76**(3A), 128-35
88. Bowden, R. A., Sayersm, F. N., Newton, B., Banaji, M., Thomas, E. D. and Meyers, J. D.

(1986). Cytomegalovirus immune globulin and seronegative blood products to prevent primary cytomegalovirus infection after marrow-transplant. *N. Engl. J. Med.*, **314**, 1006-10

89. Sulliger, J., Imbach, P., Barandun, S., Gugler, E., Hirt, A., Luthy, A., Rossi, E., Tonz, O. and Wagner, H. P. (1984). Varicella and herpes zoster in immune suppressed children: preliminary results of treatment with intravenous immunoglobulin. *Helv. Paediatr Acta*, **39**, 63-70

90. Gupta, A., Novick, B. E. and Rubinstein, A. (1986). Restoration of suppressor T-cell functions in children with AIDS following intravenous gammaglobulin treatment. *Am. J. Dis. Child.*, **140**(2), 143-6

91. Silverman, B. A. and Rubinstein, A. (1985). Serum lactate dehydrogenase levels in adults and children with acquired immune deficiency syndrome (AIDS) and AIDS-related complex: possible indicator of B cell lymphoproliferation and disease activity. Effect of intravenous gammaglobulin on enzyme levels. *Am. J. Med.*, **78**(5), 728-36

92. Mease, P. J., Ochs, M. D. and Wedgwood, R. T. (1981). Successful treatment of echovirus meningo encephalitis and myositis-fascitis with intravenous immunoglobulin therapy in a patient with X-linked agammaglobulinemia. *N. Engl. J. Med.*, **304**, 1278-81

93. Prince, A. M., Horowitz, B. and Brotman, B. (1986). Sterilization of hepatitis and HTLV III virus by exposure to Tri(n) butyl phosphate and sodium cholate. *Lancet*, **1**, 706-10

4
Chronic Herpes Virus Infections

D. H. CRAWFORD AND J. G. P. SISSONS

INTRODUCTION

Herpes viruses are DNA viruses, and if it is assumed that they all have a common ancestor, their current structural divergence suggests a long history of co-evolution with their particular host species over some 400 million years. Over this period of time they have become particularly well-adapted parasites and have established a unique relationship with their natural hosts. Thus, although primary infection is regularly accompanied by the appearance of neutralizing antibodies in the infected host, the virus is not completely eliminated from the body but persists in a 'latent' form in host tissues for the remainder of the host's life, usually without harmful effect. This benign and relatively stable co-existence between herpes viruses and their natural hosts is obviously advantageous for the survival of herpes viruses as a group. Occasional reactivations of the latent infection, with renewed production of infectious virus, sometimes accompanied by episodic disease, can occur at any time throughout the life of the infected host, and disruption of the host/virus balance leading to severe disease may occur in the immunocompromised host.

Herpes viruses can infect cells in different ways, the outcome of any one virus–cell interaction being dependent upon the identity of the virus, the identity of the cell and the environment in which the infection occurs. The different types of infection can be summarized as follows:

(1) Productive infection, with the release of viral progeny and cell death;

(2) Non-productive infection, in which the viral genome may be latent, but capable of activation into productive infection, or expressed to cause malignant transformation of the cell, but again capable of activation into productive infection.

Recently herpes viruses have been classified into three subgroups (α, β, γ) on the basis of the biological and clinical characteristics of the infection, and these can be correlated with the base composition (G-C content) of the viral genomes[1]. Thus α herpes viruses have a broad host specificity and, after an asymptomatic or mild primary infection, establish latent infection in neuronal cells. Reactivation of this infection leads to replication of the virus in the epithelial cell surfaces supplied by the affected neurons to produce a clinical lesion. Human herpes simplex viruses 1 and 2 (HSV 1 and 2) and varicella zoster virus ((VZV) are examples of herpes viruses which generally have a high genomic G-C content of 60–70%. γ herpes viruses, which include the Epstein-Barr (EB) virus, have a narrow host range, with primary infection being either asymptomatic or manifest as a mononucleosis syndrome. These viruses replicate in epithelial cells and lymphocytes, and latency is established in the latter cell type. γ herpes viruses are aetiologically associated with tumours, usually of lymphoid cells, and the G-C content of the genome is generally low. β herpes viruses, which include the cytomegaloviruses (CMV), form an intermediate group, in which primary infection may again be asymptomatic or manifest as a mononucleosis syndrome. CMV will be discussed later in this Chapter. These viruses are extremely species specific, and replicate in a variety of cell types including fibroblasts and epithelial cells. The site of latency is unknown.

EPSTEIN–BARR VIRUS

EB virus is unusual among the herpes virus family in being associated with several different disease states (Table 4.1). It is the direct aetiological agent of

Table 4.1 EB virus-associated diseases

Association	Disease	References
Causative agent	Infectious mononucleosis	2
Aetiologically associated with	Burkitt's lymphoma	4, 65
	Nasopharyngeal carcinoma	3, 81
	Lymphoproliferative disease in immunosuppressed	5
	X-linked lymphoproliferative syndrome	77
	Chronic infectious mononucleosis	82
	? recurrent parotitis	83
	? chronic interstitial pneumonitis in AIDS infants	84
	? cryptogenic fibrosing alveolitis	85
	? hairy leukoplakia in AIDS patients	86
Abnormal EBV serology	malignant lymphoma and leukaemia, e.g. Hodgkin's disease autoimmune diseases e.g. rheumatoid arthritis, systemic lupus erythematosis congenital immunodeficiencies, e.g. ataxia telangiectasia acquired immunodeficiencies, e.g. transplant recipients, AIDS	48

infectious mononucleosis (IM)[2], whereas in two geographically restricted tumours, anaplastic nasopharyngeal carcinoma[3] and African Burkitt's lymphoma[4], it acts as one factor in a complex series of events which lead to eventual malignant disease. EB virus has more recently been implicated in the aetiology of lymphoproliferative disorders in immunocompromised individuals[5], in some cases of chronic IM[6], and in the rapidly fatal acute IM which develops in the X-linked or sporadic lymphoproliferative syndrome (LPS)[7,8].

Virology

EB virus is a large virus with a molecular weight of around 100 million daltons. The virion DNA, which is double stranded and linear, is approximately 170 kb long, and the complete genome has recently been sequenced[9]. This is surrounded by an icosahedral capsid which consists of 162 triangular capsomeres and is 100 nm in diameter. This is in turn surrounded by a lipid envelope which is acquired by the budding of the immature particle through the cell surface membrane of the infected cell, and is essential for infectivity. EB virus infects cells by utilizing the CD21 antigen as a cell surface receptor for attachment[10]. This antigen, which is expressed on mature B lymphocytes[11] and some epithelial cells[12], also acts as the receptor for the C3d complement component (CR2) in the former cell type. These two cell types can be infected by the virus both *in vivo* and *in vitro*, but the outcome of their infection differs markedly.

Infection of B lymphocytes

Although all mature B lymphocytes bind and internalize EB virus particles[13], only a small percentage become activated by this process[14]. Some infected B cells are polyclonally activated in a T cell-independent manner[15] and are induced to terminally differentiate into Ig secreting plasma cells which are short lived[16]. Others become immortalized to yield continuously growing lymphoblastoid cell lines (LCL)[17]. These two populations can be distinguished by the surface expression of CD23, a B cell activation antigen[18], early after infection on those cells destined to become immortalized[19]. The CD23 molecule, which has recently been shown to be secreted by the cells, acts as an autostimulatory growth factor[20], several of which have been described as being necessary for the continued proliferation of LCL[21,22].

Within LCL only a small minority of cells are lytically infected and show expression of the EB viral early antigen (diffuse (D) and restricted (R) components) and capsid antigen complexes, with production of viral progeny[23] and cell death (Figure 4.1). In the majority of cells the infectious cycle appears to be halted at a stage of viral antigen expression which is compatible with continued cell proliferation. In these cells the viral genome is carried as multiple episomal, circular DNA molecules in the host cell nucleus which replicate with the host cell DNA and are transferred to each daughter cell, leaving the viral genome copy number constant. This so-called latent infection can be identified at the protein level by the expression of the EB

63

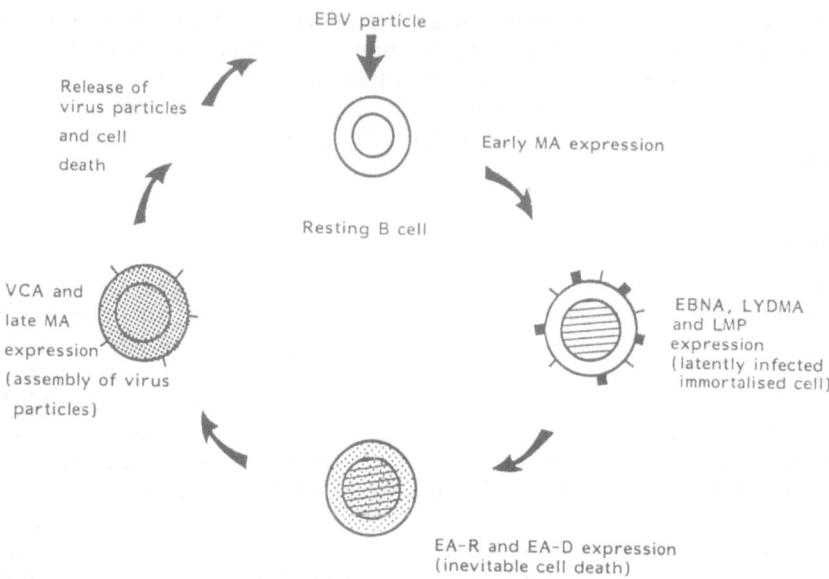

EB VIRUS LYTIC CYCLE

EBV particle

Release of virus particles and cell death

Early MA expression

Resting B cell

VCA and late MA expression (assembly of virus particles)

EBNA, LYDMA and LMP expression (latently infected immortalised cell)

EA-R and EA-D expression (inevitable cell death)

MA = Membrane antigen
EBNA = EB viral nuclear antigen
LYDMA = Lymphocyte detected membrane antigen
LMP = Latent membrane protein
EA-R = Early antigen-restricted
EA-D = Early antigen-diffuse
VCA = Viral capsid antigen

Figure 4.1 EB virus lytic cycle showing EB virus-coded antigen expression in an infected B cell

viral nuclear antigen complex (EBNA)[24] and the latent membrane protein (LMP)[25] (Figure 4.1). EBNA is now known to be a complex of at least five nuclear antigens (EBNA 1–5) of which EBNA 1 is necessary for the maintenance of the plasmid EBV DNA[26] and EBNA 2 may be important in the immortalization process. LMP, which may act as a growth factor receptor, has recently been shown to growth transform rodent cells in culture[27].

The type of infection established by EB virus in B lymphocytes *in vivo* is unknown, but it is assumed to be similar to an *in vitro* latent type of infection with long-lived memory B cells carrying the viral genome in a relatively stable manner. In contrast, Burkitt's lymphoma B cells represent a population of EB virus genome-carrying, malignantly-transformed cells which show a variable and restricted pattern of latent gene expression[28] (see later).

Infection of epithelial cells

EB virus infection of cultured squamous epithelial cells leads to a lytic infection in a small proportion of cells[29]; *in vitro* immortalization of this cell type by natural infection has not yet been achieved. Lytically infected epithelial cells have been recovered from the oropharynx[30] and uterine cervix[31] of infected individuals but no latent or non-permissive infection has been identified in normal epithelium although EB virus carrying epithelial cells form the malignant cell population in anaplastic nasopharyngeal carcinoma[32]. Although these cells have been relatively poorly studied, a restricted form of gene expression with EBNA but no lytic infection is known to exist in these cells.

The reasons for the diverse types of interaction between EB virus and B lymphocytes and epithelial cells both *in vivo* and *in vitro* are unknown, but recent evidence suggests an association with the stage of differentiation of the cell. Thus in general, mature squamous epithelial cells support the replication of DNA viruses better than the immature basal cell[33], and EB virus replication in LCL is restricted to the more mature plasmacytoid B cells[34].

Primary infection with EB virus

Epidemiology

In common with other herpes viruses in man and in animals, EB virus infects most individuals subclinically during childhood, resulting in over 90% seropositivity in adults worldwide[35]. Following primary infection the virus maintains a life-long infection in the host which is usually harmless. However, if primary infection is delayed until adolescence or early adult life, around 50% of cases are clinically manifest as IM[36]. This disease is more common in the upper socioeconomic groups and in the western world because these individuals are relatively protected from infection during childhood. The reason for the age restriction in IM is unknown, but the size of the viral dose may be an important factor. Furthermore, since the virus is probably spread by oral and perhaps sexual contact, the changing social habits at the time of adolescence may account for this finding.

During primary infection the virus usually enters the body via the mouth, and sets up a productive infection in squamous epithelial cells lining the throat, from which site B lymphocytes in the lymphoid tissue of Waldyer's ring probably become secondarily infected. Thus, early in the disease, lytically infected, desquamated epithelial cells[30], as well as infectious viral particles[37], can be recovered from throat washings, and a few EBNA positive B lymphocytes can be found in the circulation[38]. Recently, lytically infected epithelial cells and infectious virus have been recovered from the uterine cervix of two IM patients[31], but whether IM can result from primary infection of the genitourinary tract remains to be elucidated.

Clinical features

IM is characterized by fever, fatigue, pharyngitis, lymphadenopathy and

Table 4.2 EB virus-specific antibody patterns in normal and disease states

Antigen	Ig class	Normal seros=+	Normal sero-	Acute IM	X-LPS	X-LPS carrier	BL	NPC	Immunosuppr.	Chronic IM
VCA	M	-	-	+	+ in acute disease	-	-	-	-	+ or -
	G	+	-	+ raised 60–80%+	+	+ raised	+ raised	+ raised	+ raised	+ raised
	A	- or weak +	-	+	+	?	-	+ raised	?	?
EA-D	G	-	-	+	+	+	-	+	-	-
	A	-	-	-	?	?	-	+	-	-
EA-R	G	-	-	-	?	?	+	- or weak +	+	+
MA	G	+ weak	-	+	?	?	+ often	+	?	=
EBNA 1	M	-	-	+	-	-	-	-	-	?
	G	+	-	-	low or absent	low	+	+	low or absent	-
EBNA 2	G	- or	-	+	?	?	?	?	?	+

splenomegaly and, by the time of onset of clinical symptoms, both the humoral and cell-mediated arms of the immune response to the viral infection can be detected. The antibody response is characterized by the presence of IgM antibodies to the viral capsid antigen (VCA) and rising titres of IgG anti-VCA and early antigen (EA) diffuse component, (Table 4.2 and Figure 4.2). Recently IgM antibodies to EBNA 1[39] and IgG anti-EBNA 2 antibodies[40] have also been detected during acute IM. IgG antibodies to EBNA 1 become detectable during the convalescent period[40]. The laboratory diagnosis is based on the findings of a positive heterophil antibody, as detected by the monospot or Paul Bunnell tests, and an atypical lymphocytosis which gives the disease its name. These atypical cells are CD8-positive T lymphocytes[41], which mainly exhibit unrestricted cytotoxic[42] and suppressor cell activities[43], although an EB virus-specific component has recently been recognized[44]. Complete recovery from IM occurs in the vast majority of patients in 1–6 months.

EB virus infection in normal seropositive individuals

Following primary infection the virus remains in the body and can be detected in throat washings[37] and a few circulating B lymphocytes which give rise to spontaneous LCL in culture[45]. Recently, virus replication has been detected in the uterine cervical epithelium of two seropositive individuals

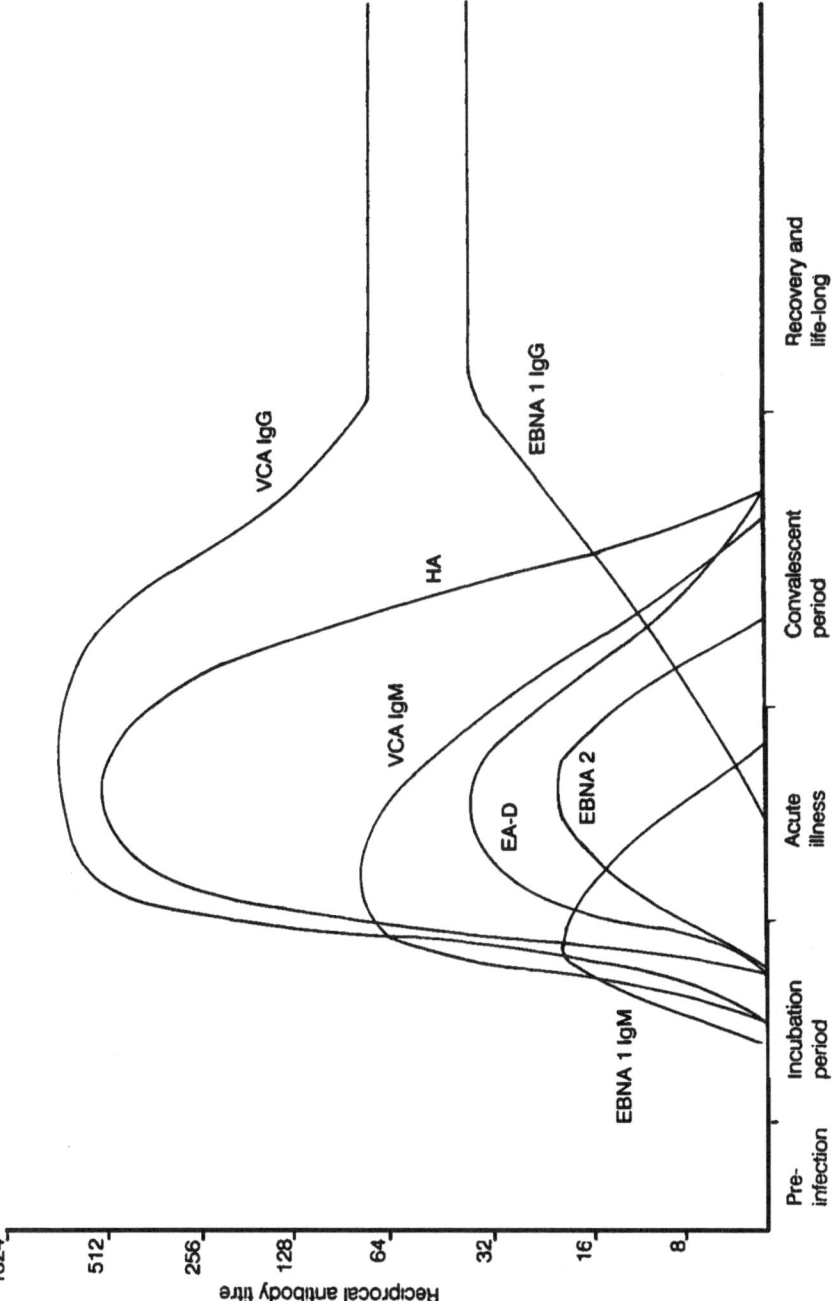

Figure 4.2 Typical EB virus specific antibody titres before, during and after acute infectious mononucleosis. H. A. = heterophil antibody

attending a sexually transmitted disease clinic for other infections[31]. This finding indicates that squamous epithelia other than that of the oropharynx can act as a site of persistence for EB virus; a similar site in the male genitourinary tract is being sought.

Humoral immune mechanisms

Following primary infection, IgG anti-VCA antibodies fall and IgG anti-EBNA 1 antibodies rise to plateau levels and persist for life, while IgG anti-EA and anti-EBNA 2 antibodies generally become undetectable (Table 4.2). These serological changes from the profile of acute IM to that of a normal seropositive individual may take up to 1 year to be completed. Antibodies to the membrane antigen complex (gp 340/220) (MA), which is present on the viral envelope and on infected B cells, neutralize viral infectivity by agglutinating virus particles. These antibodies have also been shown to mediate antibody-dependent cell cytotoxicity, so eliminating infected cells[46].

Cellular immune mechanisms

EB virus-specific, HLA restricted, CD8-positive cytotoxic memory T lymphocytes become readily detectable in the circulation during the convalescent phase of IM. These T cells were first demonstrated by their ability to cause regression of proliferating foci of EBNA-positive autologous B lymphocytes in cultures of infected peripheral blood mononuclear cells from normal seropositive individuals[47], and this regression phenomenon has since formed the basis of the regression assay which has been used to detect the presence of a specific cell-mediated immune response to EB virus in various patient groups. These T lymphocytes can be grown in long-term culture and cloned; however their antigenic specificity has not yet been determined. The putative EB virus-coded antigen(s) recognized is therefore operationally termed the lymphocyte-detected membrane antigen (LYDMA) (Figure 4.1).

This immune pattern is seen in all healthy seropositive individuals (80–90% of adults worldwide) regardless of how their primary infection was manifest, and persists for life. It is generally assumed that memory cytotoxic T cells in combination with neutralizing antibodies to MA control the persistent viral infection, so that in normal individuals a balance exists between the levels of virus replication and the immune response.

EB virus infection in immunocompromised individuals

A latent EB virus infection is reactivated in most EB virus seropositive individuals whose cell-mediated immune mechanisms have been suppressed by drugs or disease. This is manifest as increased levels of oropharyngeal virus replication, increased numbers of circulating EB virus-carrying B lymphocytes and an altered profile of antibodies to EB viral antigens (Table 4.2)[48]. These changes can be regularly found in congenital and acquired immunodeficiency states, autoimmune diseases, Hodgkin's disease, as well as with iatrogenic immunosuppression following organ transplantation (Table 4.1). In some cases this is accompanied by low or undetectable levels of circulating EB virus-specific cytotoxic T cells as detected by the regression assay[49]. These laboratory findings presumably represent a shift in the virus/host balance towards increased viral replication; however, in the majority of individuals an adequate level of control must exist, perhaps by antibody-mediated or non-specific immune mechanisms, since no symptoms occur. In a few individuals, however, lymphoproliferative lesions or lymphoma develop. Most of the studies on these lesions have been undertaken on renal transplant recipients in whom it has been known for many years that an increased incidence of lymphoma and lymphoproliferative diseases occurs[50]. Many of these have been shown to be EB virus-related, in that the cells express EBNA[51] (Figure 4.3) and/or contain EB viral DNA[52]. The incidence of these lymphoproliferative lesions was increased by cyclosporin A treatment in combination with other immunosuppressive drugs, in particular in cardiac transplant recipients[53]. Using clinical, histological, immunological and cytogenetic criteria the spectrum of lymphoproliferative diseases can be categorized into three groups of increasing malignant potential[52] (Table 4.3). Patients in groups 1 and 2 present clinically with a mononucleosis-like illness, often occurring early after transplant in young adults. The B lymphocyte proliferation is polyclonal, with the histological picture of a B lymphocyte

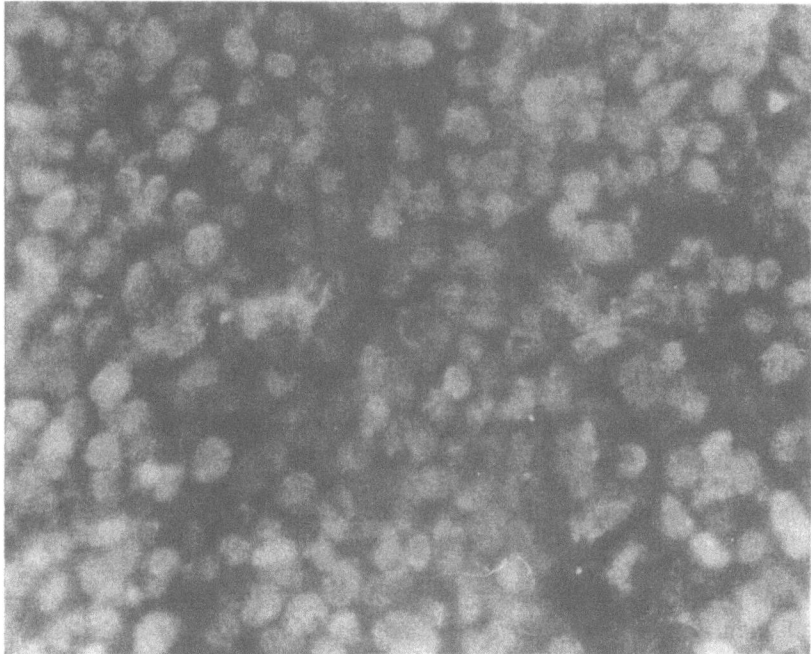

Figure 4.3 Photomicrograph of a B cell lymphoma from a renal transplant recipient. Cells are stained for the EB viral nuclear antigen complex by anticomplementary immunofluorescence and show bright nuclear fluorescence

Table 4.3 EBV-associated lymphoproliferative disease in transplant recipients

	Group 1	Group 2	Group 3
Clinical	IM like	IM like	solid tumour
Histology	B cell hyperplasia	polymorphic B cell lymphoma	polymorphic B cell lymphoma
Immunology	polyclonal	polyclonal	monoclonal
Cytogenetics	normal	clonal abnormalities in some cells	clonal abnormalities
Designation	benign	early malignant transformation	malignant lymphoma
Therapy	acyclovir	stop immunosuppression acyclovir (may fail)	lymphoma treatment

hyperplasia with a normal karyotype in group 1 and a polymorphic B cell lymphoma with clonal cytogenetic abnormalities in group 2. Patients in group 3 present with localized tumour masses, often in the central nervous system and/or gastrointestinal tract. These may occur at any time after transplantation and tend to occur in older individuals. The B cell proliferations are monoclonal, polymorphic lymphoma, and show clonal cytogenetic abnormalities. These cytogenetic abnormalities and variable and are not those characteristically found in Burkitt's lymphoma (BL) (see later). Studies of the EB viral antibody profiles in these patients show that around one third of patients presenting with a mononucleosis-like illness have a primary EB virus infection whereas the remainder in this group, and those with solid tumours, usually show a reactivated or normal antibody pattern. The three categories of disease suggest that progression from 1 to 3 may occur, and this has been documented in some cases[54].

The overall mortality without treatment exceeds 80%; however, for those patients with polyclonal lesions regression has been reported with a reduction in immunosuppressive therapy alone, or in combination with the drug acyclovir[54]. Acyclovir inhibits EB viral replication by blocking EBV DNA polymerase activity, but has no effect on the proliferation of latently infected cells *in vitro*[55]. This finding suggests that at the polyclonal stage of the disease viral replication is essential for tumour progression, and since very few, if any, of the B cells within the lesions are replicating virus, it may be that viral replication in epithelial cells, with a constant supply of secondarily infected B cells, is a necessary link in the progression of the disease. Standard lymphoma chemotherapy is essential, although not very effective, for those patients with monoclonal tumours.

This spectrum of lymphoproliferative diseases which have been studied in transplant recipients is probably similar to that occurring in other immune deficiency states, where the numbers of patients are too low to undertake detailed studies. However, some of the tumours described in AIDS patients resemble BL in that they are monoclonal tumours with the characteristic translocations involving the c-myc and immunoglobulin gene loci (see later).

Fatal infectious mononucleosis

Fatal IM is very rare, accounting for around 30 deaths per year in the USA, of which about half are sporadic cases, and half follow an X-linked pattern of inheritance – known as the X-linked lymphoproliferative syndrome (XLPS, formerly Duncan's syndrome). This disease is characterized by an abnormal response to primary EB virus infection in 50% of boys in families carrying the genetic abnormality[7]. It is rapidly fatal in most cases, but may progress to a chronic phase in which hypogammaglobulinaemia, aplastic anaemia and lymphoproliferative lesions including malignant lymphoma occur[56]. Defects in the EB virus-specific immune response described in these patients include an absence of antibodies to EBNA, and a reduced activity of EB virus-specific memory T lymphocytes[57]. In one case where the *in vivo*-infected B cells have been studied, a resistance to killing by EB virus-specific cytotoxic T cells has been noted[58]. These three findings may be linked, since if the B lymphocytes do not express the virus-coded antigens necessary for T cell recognition then no T cells would be activated and no memory cells develop. Similarly, if no B lymphocytes are lysed then the EBNA complex, as an intracellular antigen, may not stimulate the humoral arm of the immune response. Non-specific immune abnormalities described in XLPS include poor natural killer cell activity and a deficient IgM to IgG class switch[57].

Several immunodeficiency states of both cellular and humoral types map to the X chromosome, but so far the exact location and function of the putative XLPS gene have not been determined. This immunodeficiency is unique in being disease-specific, since these children apparently respond normally to other infections, including those of the other herpes viruses. XLPS carriers can usually be identified in a family by a reactivated type of EB virus-specific antibody profile (Table 4.2)

Chronic infectious mononucleosis

In a minority of cases of IM the disease may persist for over 1 year with chronic or recurrent symptoms. There is no universally recognized definition of chronic IM, and cases have even been described which lack a history of an acute episode[59]. Patients can roughly be divided into two groups (G. Miller, personal communication), although some overlap does occur.

The fatigue syndrome

This is a relatively mild syndrome of fatigue, fever, sore throat, malaise, myalgia and lymphadenopathy which shows a female preponderance and an age range of 20–30 years. No haematological or serological abnormalities occur, and its association with EB virus is therefore tenuous.

The severe form

In this syndrome there are persistent symptoms as described for the fatigue syndrome with some or all of the following findings: anaemia, leukopenia, thrombocytopenia, hypogammaglobulinaemia, hepatomegaly, splenomegaly, uveitis, pneumonitis[60]. Serological findings reflect those found in acute IM and include a rise in IgG anti-VCA, a reappearance of anti-EA (R>D) with or without anti-VCA IgM and heterophile antibody[61,62]. Antibodies to EBNA 1 are low or absent, but anti-EBNA 2 antibodies reappear[40] (Table 4.2). Cellular abnormalities described include the absence of detectable EB virus-specific cytotoxic T cells[63] and high suppressor cell activity[58]. These findings suggest a defect in the evolution of cell-mediated immunity to EB virus following acute IM resulting in the persistence of the immune profile and clinical symptoms seen in the acute disease.

Chronic IM is a long-lasting debilitating disease which, although apparently not life threatening, can severely disrupt a normal life style. There is no known beneficial therapy, although in some cases acyclovir has been used to successfully relieve symptoms[60]. This would suggest that the symptoms may be caused, at least in part, by excessive viral replication *in vivo*.

Burkitt's lymphoma

Burkitt's lymphoma is a monoclonal tumour of B lymphocytes which is the commonest tumour in children aged 5–10 years in Equatorial Africa, where it was first recognized by Denis Burkitt in 1958[64]. He described a rapidly-growing, geographically restricted multicentric tumour in children, commonly involving the jaw.

Pathogenesis of BL

Association with EB virus Following the initial description of BL, which suggested an infectious aetiological agent, EB virus was isolated from cultured BL cells[65]. The virus has subsequently been shown to be aetiologically associated with the tumour by the following experimental data:

(1) EB viral antigens (MA and EBNA) and/or EB viral DNA are found in the tumour cells in around 97% of African BL[4], and cell lines grown from the tumour cells express viral antigens and produce infectious EB virus particles.

Recent studies on viral gene expression in BL tumours and their derived cell lines have revealed a variable and restricted pattern of latent gene expression. EBNA 1 is expressed in all cells but EBNA 2 expression may be variant or absent[28]. Thus two variants have been described which differ at the EBNA 2 gene locus (2A and 2B) and which code for different proteins[66]. Alternatively, the EBNA 2 gene may be deleted[67]. LMP may also be unexpressed in BL cells, but this is not reflected by deletions at the DNA level[28]. Further analysis has shown that both the cellular and viral gene expression of BL cells alters with growth in culture to become more like the latent gene expression pattern seen in LCL. The significance of these findings is at present unclear.

(2) Antibody titres to the EB viral capsid antigen show an 8–10 times higher

geometric mean titre in African BL children than in a matched control group[4]. Antibody levels vary with tumour growth and can predict the outcome of the disease. Thus high levels of anti-MA antibody and low levels of anti-EA(R) antibody correlate with a good prognosis, a fall in level of anti-MA often indicating a relapse. A prospective study on 42000 Ugandan children has shown that EB virus infection occurs months or years before the development of BL and that those children with the highest antibody titres are at the greatest risk of developing BL[68].

(3)   The oncogenic potential of the virus is suggested by its ability to immortalize B lymphocytes *in vitro*[69]. However, the lymphoblastoid cell lines established *in vitro* differ from those established from BL tumour tissue which represent transformed cells of the malignant phenotype (see later).

(4)   EB virus has been shown to induce B cell tumours in subhuman primates such as cotton top tamarins[70]. These tumours, although of B cell origin, differ from BL in often being polyclonal or oligoclonal and lacking the characteristic chromosomal translocation seen in BL (see later).

Aetiological cofactors in BL It is now generally accepted that EB virus infection is one of the steps involved in the multistep aetiology of BL, and that other important cofactors must exist which would account for the geographical restriction of the tumour. Hyperendemic malaria has been postulated as one such cofactor since its geographical distribution is almost identical to that of BL. Other evidence supporting this association comes from studies on individuals carrying the sickle cell trait. This genetic defect of the α-haemoglobin gene products against *Plasmodium falciparum* infection, and these individuals have also been shown to be protected against developing BL. Furthermore, where the incidence of malaria has fallen due to clearance of the mosquito vector the incidence of BL has also fallen.

Recent studies from the Gambia, West Africa have shown that during acute malaria the T cells which cause regression of proliferating EB virus immortalized B cells *in vitro* cannot be detected in the circulation, but reappear on recovery from the acute disease[71]. This finding suggests that recurrent attacks of malaria allow the exaggerated proliferation of EB virus carrying B cells *in vivo*, so increasing the size of the pool of potentially malignant cells.

Chromosomal translocation Cells and cell lines derived from BL tumours all show a characteristic chromosomal translocation[72]. This translocation transfers the c-myc oncogene from chromosome 8 to a position adjacent to one of the immunoglobulin gene loci on chromosomes 14 (heavy chain), 2 (κ light chain) or 22 (λ light chain)[73]. It is postulated that the translocation of this gene to an area of the B cell genome where active transcription is occurring leads to the dysregulation of the gene with its constitutive expression within the cell. Although the normal function of the c-myc protein is unknown, its expression in actively cycling cells suggests that it is necessary for continued cell proliferation. Thus its constitutive expression would allow the cells to proliferate indefinitely without maturation, differentiation or senescence. The sequence of events occurring during the evolution of a BL tumour has been much debated, but recent evidence suggests that the translocation of the c-myc gene is most likely to occur at the time of immunoglobulin gene rearrangement in the early B cell which would then be followed by virus infection[74].

Cell-mediated immunity to EB virus in BL patients Most BL patients have normal levels of circulating EB virus-specific cytotoxic T cells, and therefore a specific immune defect alone is unlikely to account for the emergence of the tumour. However, recent studies on paired cell lines from BL patients, one derived from the tumour cell and the other by *in vitro* infection of peripheral blood B cells, have shown that some BL cell lines are resistant to killing by EB virus-specific cytotoxic T cells[75]. These data suggest a mechanism by which BL tumour cells evade the cytotoxic action of immune T cells, but the reason for this resistance is not clear, and cannot at the present time be correlated with the lack of expression of any EB virus-coded antigens. Other non-specific mechanisms by which BL cells evade the immune response, such as a lack of HLA class I expression, have also been described.

It is now recognized that tumours histologically identical to BL occur worldwide at a low incidence, and although only around one third of these are EB virus-associated, all show the characteristic chromosomal translocation. These sporadic BL account for the small number (around 3%) of African BL which are EB virus-negative. Studies on the cell surface antigen expression of sporadic and endemic BL suggest their origins from B cells at different stages of maturation. Thus endemic BL cells generally have the phenotype of bone marrow B cells whereas sporadic BL has the more mature phenotype of follicular centre B cells.

Nasopharyngeal carcinoma (NPC)

This tumour occurs worldwide at low incidence, and at high incidence in Southern China where it is the commonest tumour in men and the second commonest in women. It has an intermediate incidence in the Mediterranean basin, North and East Africa, Malaysia, Iceland and Alaska. It is the undifferentiated form of the tumour which is associated with EB virus, the circumstantial evidence being similar to that of BL[3]. Thus the tumour cells contain EB viral DNA and express EBNA, viral antibody titres (particularly anti-EA (D)) are raised and increase as the tumour burden increases. The geographical restriction of the tumour may be due to a genetic predisposition since an association with certain HLA haplotypes (A2, B17, BW45, BW58) has been described. There may also be dietary cofactors involved in the aetiology of the tumour, for which smoked fish, and phorbol ester-containing herbal remedies have been suggested[76]. NPC tumour cells have not been established in culture, and so little is known about the viral/cell interaction; however, immortalizing virus has been rescued from the tumour cells and shown to have an identical genome structure to that associated with BL and IM[77].

Future perspectives

Recently work has been undertaken in the development of a vaccine which would prevent EB virus infection, and in this way, it is argued, prevent EB virus-associated tumours by breaking the chain of events necessary for their evolution[78]. The antigen chosen as a candidate vaccine is gp 340/220, the membrane antigen to which virus-neutralizing antibodies develop during natural infection. Crude membrane preparations of LCL have induced neutralizing antibodies in cotton topped tamarins, which have then resisted challenge with a tumorogenic dose of EB virus[79]. However, when purified gp 340/220 was used as the immunogen, the method of purification proved to be an important factor in the level of protection achieved, although neutralizing antibody developed in all cases[80]. These findings suggest that the cell-mediated arm of the immune response may be more important than neutralizing antibody in preventing, as well as in controlling, EB virus infection *in vivo*, and further studies in the animal model are necessary before the ideal vaccine programme can be devised.

HUMAN CYTOMEGALOVIRUS (CMV)

Virology

Cytomegalic inclusion disease in infants has been recognized for many years (since the turn of the century), although a viral aetiology was not suspected until 1920 and the virus itself was only isolated in the 1950s. The 'cytomegalic inclusion' refers to the fact that the virus produces enlargement of the cells in which it replicates, and an inclusion body in the nucleus. CMV is relatively slow growing in tissue culture, and isolation from clinical samples may take as long as 2 weeks.

Human cytomegalovirus has the typical virion structure and electron microscopic appearances of a herpes virus. It is classed as a β herpes virus – although many species have cytomegaloviruses, they are species specific: thus human CMV will only productively infect human cells and cannot be studied experimentally in animal models. CMV has the largest genome of all the herpes viruses (235 kb) and this will soon have been completely sequenced. The virus DNA comprises a long and short unique sequence (Ul and Us) each flanked by terminal repeat sequences inverted with respect to each other – this arrangement allows for four isomeric forms of the virus DNA (Figures 4.4 and 4.5). As with other herpes viruses, three classes of viral genes and proteins are recognized – the immediate early (IE) genes are the first transcribed, within hours of infection, followed by the early (E) genes and the late (L) genes. Expression of these three classes of viral genes is tightly regulated within the infected cell, with expression of one set of genes being prerequisite for, and triggering, expression of the next. The late genes are the only ones whose products are structural components of the virus particle – the IE and E gene products are only found in infected cells[87].

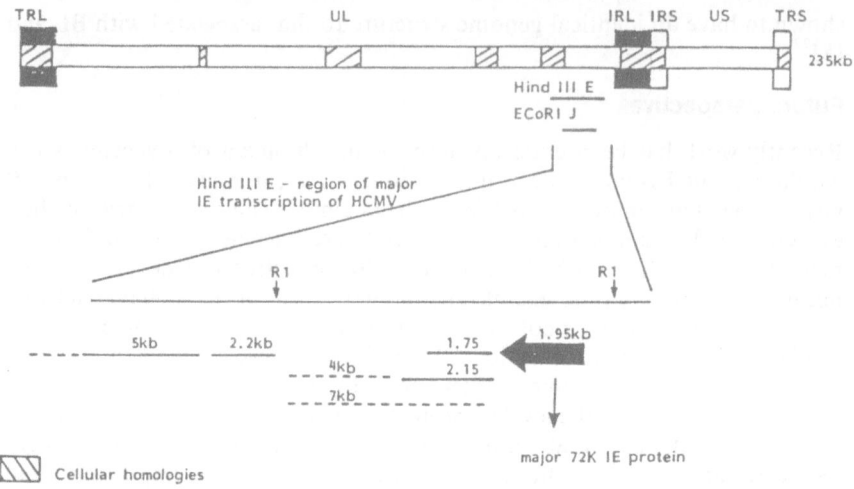

Figure 4.4 Genome structure of HCMV and RNA transcripts from the region of immediate early transcription

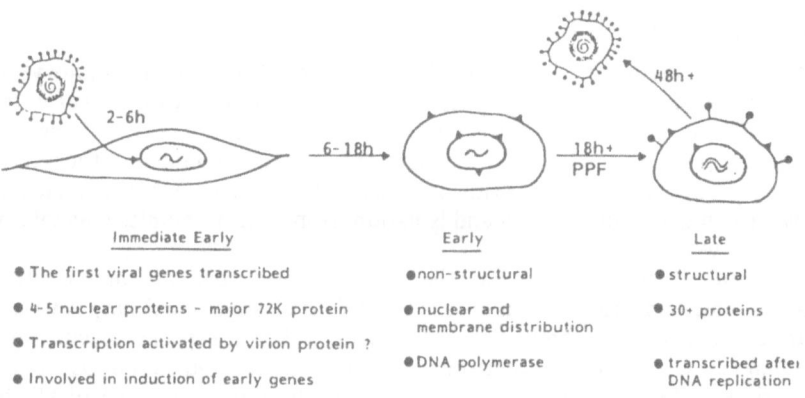

Figure 4.5 Human cytomegalovirus – gene expression and protein synthesis. See text for further details

Any detailed consideration of the molecular biology of CMV is beyond the scope of this chapter but some aspects are pertinent to the immunology. The sequence of events during productive infection is approximately as follows. Whether or not expression of the immediate early genes occurs depends on the cell infected and probably requires specific transcription factors which are present only in certain cells. In addition, proteins on the virus particle may themselves transactivate expression of the immediate early genes – that is, a structural protein can initiate transcription in *trans* from the immediate early promoter; this is unequivocally established for herpes simplex but is less certain for CMV. CMV has about six immediate early genes. The most abundant immediate early RNA transcript codes for a 72 kDa nuclear protein, the major immediate early protein. The role of all these immediate early proteins is uncertain but they transactivate the early genes, and may also transactivate cellular genes. HCMV does not shut off host protein synthesis, unlike HSV[88]. The early gene products are incompletely characterized but some are glycoproteins and one is the virus DNA polymerase. Following expression of the early genes, DNA replication occurs and only after this are the late genes expressed and their proteins synthesized: virus assembly occurs and progeny virus particles are released. Expression of the late proteins can be prevented by treating infected cells with sodium phosphonoformate (PPF), a reversible inhibitor of the virus DNA polymerase which is used both as an experimental tool and a drug for the treatment of CMV disease.

There are around 30 proteins in the virion itself. Their functions and precise number remain uncertain. There are capsid proteins, and at least three matrix proteins including the 64-68 kDa matrix protein which is the most abundant in the virion, and at least six viral glycoproteins are described: the major glycoprotein is a 145 kDa protein showing homology with glycoprotein B of HSV[89].

The only cell fully permissive for CMV replication *in vitro* is the diploid fibroblast; limited expression of CMV has been reported in a number of other cell types including endothelial cells, epithelial cells, bone marrow, lymphoid cells and lymphoblastoid cell lines. However, all these latter reports require further confirmation and study. The cell surface receptor for CMV is quite unknown (unlike that for EBV) and so whether receptor-determined tropism is the reason for this restriction of CMV replication is likewise unknown. One interesting aspect which has been studied *in vitro* is that CMV can reportedly infect teratoma cell lines but not even the IE genes are expressed. However, when these cell lines are induced to differentiate (with retinoic acid) virus gene expression occurs and they then become permissive for virus replication[90]. The possibility that CMV could infect a cell but only replicate when that cell differentiates is an attractive concept, but further work is needed to explain the mechanism.

Epidemiology

CMV is widely distributed in human populations, like the other herpes viruses. Taking seropositivity (usually by the relatively crude complement fixation text) as the index of infection, the following pattern emerges. Seropositivity in adult populations approaches 100% in most third world countries, but is about 40-60% in developed countries. Seroconversion occurs earlier in developing countries so that around 80-90% of children in Melanesia and Tanzania were seropositive by 5-6 years compared to 5-30% in the USA. The number of seropositive people progressively increases with age. Within developed countries CMV infection is more prevalent in both lower socioeconomic and sexually promiscuous groups. From the epidemiology, and from what is known of the biology of CMV, transmission of virus is presumed to occur by contact with secretions (including saliva, breast milk, semen and cervical secretions) which contain CMV.

Sites of persistence of CMV

Knowing where the virus persists is a fundamental prerequisite to understanding its biology. However, despite considerable speculation and unsubstantiated observation, there is remarkably little firm information in this area. It seems fairly certain that CMV must persist in the salivary gland (by analogy with the mouse, and because CMV is intermittently shed in saliva) and the kidney or lower urinary tract epithelium (because CMV is intermittently excreted in the urine). It is also possible that CMV may persist in the epithelial cells in the gut, where it produces clinical problems in immunosuppressed patients. Even for these, highly likely, sites definitive evidence is lacking. Probably the best method for detecting persistent CMV would be sensitive *in situ* hybridization assays, but such assays have only just begun to be applied to normal seropositive CMV carriers, with a view to determining sites of virus persistence. The situation is particularly confused when we come to the question of whether CMV persists in cells of the peripheral blood. There is no doubt that CMV can be transmitted by blood transfusion but which cell is responsible is uncertain. Application of *in situ* hybridization to peripheral blood mononuclear cells from normal seropositive subjects has been reported to show immediate early RNA transcripts in up to 2% of cells, mainly T4$^+$ lymphocytes and monocytes[91]. However, this figure is almost certainly too high, and these same workers and ourselves have subsequently found that most seropositive subjects show only the occasional positive cell in the *in situ* assay. Although serial studies on the same subjects may show fluctuations in the number of positive cells, this averages around 0.002%. During overt clinical CMV infection virus can be isolated from blood relatively frequently, especially from buffy coat; however, the frequency of lymphocytes and monocytes scoring positive in the *in situ* assay during clinically overt infection is not very much greater than in asymptomatic carriers (around 0.01–0.1%). There is a suggestion both from virus isolation studies and dot blot hybridization, that CMV may be present in neutrophils during overt infection. This again needs confirming as neutrophils seem an intrinsically improbable site for the virus to persist in view of their short half-life[92].

Turning to the question of whether cell lines of lymphoid or monocytic lineage can be infected *in vitro*, we find similar uncertainties. Certainly CMV does not usually replicate in fresh peripheral blood mononuclear cells, or in lymphoid or monocytic cell lines, but it has been reported that expression of CMV IE genes (as detected by monoclonal antibodies against the major IE protein) may occur in a small proportion (0.1% or less) of such cells infected *in vitro*. Further difficulty arises because it has been reported that even this limited gene expression is only seen if recent clinical isolates of CMV are used[93, 94] (as opposed to the laboratory strains such as AD169 which have been serially passaged in fibroblasts for years).

Taking such evidence as there is, a reasonable summary of current information would be that CMV may well be carried in a very small proportion (not more than 1 in 1000–5000 cells) of peripheral blood mononuclear cells, but there is no evidence any such cell is a normal site of replication. Nevertheless, even such a very low frequency of cells carrying CMV could transmit infection by blood transfusion.

Functional effects of CMV on the immune response

It is a widely held view that CMV infection *in vivo* is itself capable of producing immunosuppression as evidenced by its association with other opportunistic infections[95]. This is inevitably somewhat anecdotal. Obviously CMV disease itself normally occurs in the context of pre-existing immunosuppression. However, there is some experimental evidence to support the idea that CMV may be immunosuppressive. Thus it has been reported that peripheral blood mononuclear cells from patients with primary CMV infection and CMV mononucleosis do not show a normal proliferative response to mitogens, and this lack of proliferation has been attributed to a suppressive effect mediated by adherent cells, monocytes in particular[96, 97]. It seems quite possible that the increased numbers of CD8+ cells present in peripheral blood during active CMV infection may account for some of these suppressive effects.

Other studies have been based on infecting cells with CMV *in vitro*. Experimental infection of *normal* peripheral blood mononuclear cells with CMV *in vitro* has been reported to produce suppression of responses to mitogens (Con A and PHA)[97]. Experimental infection of monocytes has been reported to abrogate IL-1 release by the cells[98]. Suppressive effects of CMV on the effector function of cytotoxic cells have also been described: infection of natural killer cells *in vitro* has been reported to suppress their cytotoxic activity[99]. There are two problems with these *in vitro* observations. The first is that it is somewhat difficult to attribute these *in vitro* suppressive effects to direct infection by CMV when (as just discussed) there is such very limited evidence of virus infection or virus gene expression in the cells (monocytes and lymphocytes) involved. The second is that some of these effects could be explained by mycoplasma contamination of the CMV used in the studies. It is clear that mycoplasma can produce artefacts, such as diminishing [3H] thymidine incorporation or inhibiting cell proliferation. In our own hands, it is difficult to reproduce most of these suppressive effects attributed to CMV *in vitro* if virus isolates shown to be free of mycoplasmas are used. Thus the precise mechanisms for any immunosuppressive effects of CMV, and the relative contributions of direct infection of immunocompetent cells and indirect induced changes in cell populations, remain to be determined.

The immune response against CMV

Circumstantial evidence suggests that, as with other herpes viruses, the major component of the immune response involved in maintaining the virus host balance in normal subjects is the T cell response. Because of the comparative rarity with which primary CMV infection is recognized, there has been little study on the nature of the T cell response during CMV mononucleosis. However, the specificity of memory CMV specific T cells in the peripheral blood of asymptomatic virus carriers has been analysed and it has been shown that classical cytotoxic cells (Tc) can be demonstrated, restricted by class I MHC antigens[100]. It appears that the majority of these CMV specific Tc are directed against determinants expressed at immediate early or early times, as evidenced by the fact that cells treated with phosphonoformate are lysed. It appears from our own studies using limiting dilution analysis, that the majority of CMV specific Tc precursors in peripheral blood are directed towards immediate early antigens[101]. Recombinant vaccinia viruses expressing the CMV major immediate early gene and glycoprotein B have been constructed, and are now being used to analyse the specificity of CMV Tc. Initial results suggest that the major immediate early protein itself is a major target for Tc, whilst a smaller proportion (about 20%) of CMV specific Tc precursors recognize cells infected with a glycoprotein B vaccinia recombinant[101]. If the predominant specificity of CMV specific cytotoxic T cells is for this major IE protein, which is a nuclear protein, this would be a further example of virus specific Tc recognizing predominantly intracellular proteins[102]. This human work correlates with work on murine CMV (MCMV) infection by Reddehase, Kosinowski *et al.*[103]. They have shown that during acute primary MCMV infection Tc cells from a draining lymph node comprise two distinct populations: one which recognizes MCMV infected cells expressing late antigens and another recognizing cells expressing only immediate early gene products[103]. However, during persistent MCMV infection the bulk of MCMV specific Tc precursors in spleen cells are directed towards the MCMV major immediate early protein. Transfer experiments have shown that the MCMV specific Tc population confers protection against lethal MCMV infection whereas Th (L3T4) cells do not[104].

All this work suggests the existence of a Tc surveillance system against CMV in the persistently infected human host, probably somewhat akin to that which appears to exist against EBV. The assumption would be that it is the suppression of this mechanism that predisposes to disseminated CMV disease. This is obviously speculative, just as it is in the case of EBV.

There have been a few studies on the effect of natural killer (NK) cells on CMV-infected cells *in vitro*. In one study CMV-infected cells become susceptible to NK cell killing when early antigens were expressed[105]. Of course, as with all human virus infections, an objective assessment of the role of NK cells is difficult. However, in murine CMV infection NK cells have been shown to be capable of producing resolution of infection by adoptive transfer experiments, virtually the only virus for which this has been done[106].

Antibodies are made against all classes of viral proteins – immediate early, early and late, but the role of antibody in protection against CMV is unknown. As is the case for other herpes viruses, neutralizing antibody seems more likely to be of importance in preventing primary infection than reactivation. Monoclonal antibodies have been produced against a number of CMV proteins: monoclonals against the glycoprotein designated gB have virus neutralizing activity[89], and gB may thus be one potential candidate for a CMV vaccine.

Relatively little is known of how CMV specific immunity is disturbed during clinical CMV disease. It has been reported that CMV specific cytotoxic T cell activity is detectable directly (without secondary *in vitro* stimulation) in the peripheral blood of some subjects with active CMV disease, and it has been claimed that its detection is a favourable prognostic sign. In bone marrow transplant recipients the absence of CMV specific cytotoxicity was associated with high mortality[107]. In patients with AIDS and CMV infection it has been reported that CMV specific cytotoxic T cells cannot be directly detected, but can be induced *in vitro* by treating their peripheral blood lymphocytes with exogenous IL-2 alone[108]. This could be interpreted as evidence for activated precursor cytotoxic T cells being present *in vivo*, unable to expand because of the defective IL-2 production.

Clinical presentation

Primary CMV infection

Primary CMV infection in healthy subjects is frequently asymptomatic but may be associated with a mononucleosis syndrome clinically very similar to that produced by EBV. The distinction is that patients with CMV mononucleosis do not develop heterophile antibody. Tonsillitis and pharyngitis are said to be less common than with EBV mononucleosis, and lymphadenopathy less marked. As with EBV, primary CMV infection presumably frequently goes unrecognized. Several rare clinical complications may occur with primary infection. These include hepatitis (although mildly abnormal liver function tests are much commoner), meningoencephalitis, thrombocytopenia, and intestitial pneumonitis (and perhaps Guillain–Barre syndrome). Some of these occasional complications of primary infection in normal subjects are seen as much more frequent accompaniments of CMV infection in immunosuppressed subjects. This general clinical picture of a mononucleosis syndrome occurs however primary CMV infection is acquired, whether by acquisition from casual contact, or from infection by blood transfusion[109].

Investigations during primary infection show a lymphocytosis with atypical mononuclear cells (up to 60% of total count). IgM antibody is detectable within a week of infection and IgG antibody (by complement fixation) within 2 weeks. Virus may be isolated from throat and urine. A general problem pertaining to tissue culture isolation of CMV has been that, although its distinctive cytopathic effect (CPE) is readily identifiable, it takes at least some days to develop. A number of laboratories have recently utilized monoclonal antibodies against immediate early or early antigens of CMV to detect their expression by immunofluorescence before the appearance of CPE. This means that virus can be detected within 24 hours – however, such antibodies are not yet widely available[110].

Following primary infection, CMV persistence is established and the lifelong carrier state ensues. As discussed above, however, there is still uncertainty over the sites at which CMV persists. In the case of EBV it is clear that normal asymptomatic virus carriers shed infectious virus intermittently from the oropharynx. Whether CMV is shed in urine or saliva intermittently in normal subjects is not known; however, it seems likely that it may be (and in semen and cervical secretions as well) in view of the probability that these body fluids may all be routes by which the virus is transmitted. This is not solely of academic interest as it bears on the question of whether virus excretion is evidence of 'reactivation' (by implication likely to be abnormal and pathological) or simply a normal if intermittent concomitant of the carrier state. Certainly there is no evidence that lifelong carriage of CMV is detrimental to the normal healthy host. This is in marked contrast to the situation in immunosuppressed subjects.

CMV infection in immunosuppressed subjects

Primary infection, and to a lesser extent reactivation of endogenous virus, can produce much more serious illness in subjects with pre-existing immuno-suppression. Infection is more likely to be disseminated and to produce more severe organ involvement. In fact, in the absence of satisfactory chemotherapy (see below), CMV infection is a major cause of death in bone marrow transplant recipients (together with graft versus host disease) and to a lesser but still significant extent in cardiac, liver and renal transplanta-tion[111, 112]. CMV infection is also a very common problem in patients with AIDS, and affects nearly all patients, particularly towards the end of their clinical course. In any immunosuppressed patient, primary infection tends to produce more severe manifestations than disease caused by reactivation. In this context donor organs (kidney, marrow and liver) as well as blood, are capable of transmitting infection and many units now avoid using organs or blood from CMV seropositive donors in seronegative recipients.

Although clinically significant CMV infection may be manifest as a febrile mononucleosis syndrome, just as in immunocompetent patients, organ involvement is the hallmark of more serious disease, as briefly summarized below.

Interstitial pneumonitis is the most common presentation of CMV infection in immunosuppressed subjects. There are, of course, many other causes of this picture in such patients. Other opportunistic agents such as fungi, pneumocystis and bacteria may produce pneumonitis. However, although CMV is frequently isolated in association with these agents, it is clear that it can produce severe pneumonitis in its own right. CMV pneumonitis associated with hypoxia carries a particularly bad prognosis. *Hepatitis* due to CMV may be severe in immunosuppressed subjects. There is increasing evidence that CMV may produce disease of the *gastrointestinal tract*. CMV is often detected at autopsy of immunosuppressed patients by histology of the gastrointestinal tract, and its presence there has also been detected by *in situ* hybridization – both in the absence of obvious pathology[113]. However, CMV has also been associated with ulceration of the stomach and colon, and with severe colitis; although an aetiological association is hard to prove, the impression is growing that CMV is causally associated with such lesions in many cases. For instance, in bone marrow transplantation much gut disease formerly attributed to GVHD is now thought to be CMV associated, and in patients with AIDS CMV may also produce enteritis. *Retinitis* is another serious manifestation of CMV disease. The characteristic appearances in the adult are of white necrotic areas mingled with flame-shaped haemorrhages. The disease involves the retina and pigment epithelium. The retinitis if extensive can cause permanent loss of sight, and is again common in AIDS. Isolation of virus from the eye is usually impractible, as is biopsy, and the diagnosis thus depends on the clinical appearances and concurrent isolation of CMV from another site. *Adrenalitis* due to CMV has been reported in a few AIDS patients, associated with adrenal failure. CMV has also been reported in the *brain* of AIDS patients but the extent to which it contributes to AIDS dementia or encephalitis is uncertain[114].

A rather fundamental problem raised by these protean manifestations of CMV in immunosuppressed subjects is why this apparent discrepancy exists between the very limited number of cell types in which CMV will grow *in vitro*, and the widespread distribution of affected tissues in disseminated CMV disease.

In all these situations diagnosis depends on isolation of virus in association with a clinical picture compatible with CMV disease. Primary infection may be detected by seroconversion, but CMV antibody titres are relatively little use in diagnosing CMV disease due to reactivation of endogenous virus. If virus can be isolated from blood (buffy coat) it suggests dissemination and makes it more likely that any concurrent clinical syndrome is related to CMV. There may be a lymphocytosis. One interesting fact which has emerged from studies of phenotypic markers on T cells following transplantation, is that CMV disease (and other herpes virus infections) are accompanied by an increase in the number of circulating $CD8^+$ cells. This may persist for months – the precise functional attributes of these $T8^+$ cells are unknown[115].

Involvement of CMV in graft rejection and GVHD

It has been suggested that there is a higher incidence of graft rejection in renal allograft recipients who develop CMV disease. However, this is not a consistent finding, with only some centres reporting it. Furthermore, even where an association is reported it is not clearly causal[111]. It could be for instance that the increased immunosuppression given for rejection predisposes to CMV disease. It has also been suggested that CMV may produce a distinct form of glomerulopathy in transplanted kidneys, which should be distinguished from rejection and is an indication for reduction in immunosuppressive therapy. However, the existence of this specific glomerulopathy has not been universally accepted[116].

Murine CMV has been reported to increase alloreactive responses to MHC antigens and enhance GVHD in transplanted mice[117]. However, there is no established association of CMV with GVHD in human bone marrow transplantation despite the fact that both GVHD and CMV disease are common occurrences.

A sequence of amino acid homology between the IE2 protein of CMV and a conserved region of the HLA-DR B chain has recently been described. A synthetic peptide corresponding to this sequence in the virus elicited antibody which cross-reacted with DR. This could be of considerable theoretical interest as a possible mechanistic explanation for some of the above phenomena.

Congenital CMV infection

The epidemiology of maternal and perinatal CMV infection has been studied quite extensively. CMV is excreted from the cervix and the rate of cervical shedding increases during the third trimester of pregnancy. Transmission to the neonate may thus occur during birth. Such perinatally acquired CMV infection may occur in around a third of infants born to mothers excreting CMV in the third trimester; it is characterized by viruria first detectable at 4–8 weeks after birth and is nearly always asymptomatic and not associated with any long-term damage. In a series from Alabama about 5% of all live births were associated with such perinatal CMV infection, although this figure reflects the relatively high prevalence of CMV infection in a low socioeconomic group[118, 119].

True congenital or intrauterine CMV infection is rarer and occurs in 0.5–2% of live births. A number of studies indicate that the risk of symptomatic congenital CMV infection is very much greater with primary maternal CMV infection occurring during pregnancy[108, 118]. Figures from these studies suggest that about half the infants born to mothers experiencing primary infection in pregnancy will acquire intrauterine CMV infection, and half of these will be symptomatic. Classical congenital cytomegalic inclusion disease is characterized by jaundice and hepatosplenomegaly, a petechial rash, and CNS involvement with microcephaly, cerebral calcification, chorioretinitis and inner ear involvement. However, this classical picture is the extreme and more subtle defects, particularly nerve deafness and mild intellectual impairment, may also occur. Intrauterine infection is diagnosed by viruria at birth and IgM antibody may be present in cord blood.

CMV and oncogenesis

CMV has been proposed as a candidate oncogenic virus, as have the other herpes viruses. However, there is no conclusive evidence as yet to link it definitively with any human cancer. CMV has been reported to produce transformation *in vitro*, both the whole CMV genome and fragments of the DNA. The transfection experiments using cloned restriction fragments reported that a 489 nucleotide fragment could produce transformation and yet no CMV DNA could be detected in the transformants, suggesting a role only in the initiation of transformation.

It has been suggested that CMV is associated with Kaposi's sarcoma – this was with the African endemic form, before the appearance of Kaposi's sarcoma in association with AIDS; CMV sequences detected by *in situ* hybridization were reported in the Kaposi's sarcoma lesions. However, this work was done with whole viral DNA probes. It is now realized that the CMV genome contains considerable stretches of sequence homology with mammalian cellular DNA; selection of probes which avoid these regions is therefore important to avoid artefact. More recent work using better probes in African and AIDS-associated Kaposi's sarcoma has not confirmed the presence of CMV. An association with genital cancers (prostatic and cervical carcinoma) has also been proposed but there is no hard evidence to support these claims. Further details are available in reviews[120].

Treatment

It is still the case that therapy of CMV disease is unsatisfactory. Although a number of different treatments have been tried in the past only those currently in use are discussed.

Anti-viral chemotherapy

HCMV does not code for its own thymidine kinase (Tk) and thus, not surprisingly, acyclovir is ineffective against it. However, newer nucleoside analogues which do have activity against HCMV are currently under investigation. The only one which has been clinically investigated is DHPG (9-dihydroxy propoxymethyl guanine). In initial uncontrolled trials DHPG has been reported to be of use in treating CMV disease in immunosuppressed patients. These are mainly bone marrow transplant recipients and those with AIDS[121]. However, the impression is that patients with interstitial pneumonitis show a relatively poorer response than those with other manifestations of CMV disease. In view of the high relapse rate in patients with AIDS, maintenance regimes have been devised involving administration of DHPG up to 5 times weekly on an outpatient basis. DHPG has to be administered intravenously. Its main drawback is its radiomimetic side-effects, principally bone marrow suppression, which limit its use in many patients. It was synthesized independently by four pharmaceutical companies and is available on a named patient basis in the UK from two (Wellcome and Syntex). Perhaps its main importance is that it points the way to newer synthetic nucleoside analogues which may be less toxic and more effective.

Trisodium phosphonoformate (Foscarnet) is not a nucleoside analogue but a reversible competitive inhibitor of the virus DNA polymerase. It has been used experimentally in the laboratory for many years as a tool to restrict expression of herpes virus genes in tissue culture. It prevents virus DNA replication by its inhibition of the DNA polymerase. In fact it also has activity against a number of other virus specified polymerases and is under investigation for the treatment of HIV infection and of fulminant hepatitis B. It has not been subjected to controlled trials, but is available for use on a named patient basis (Astra Pharmaceuticals). Impressions are that it does have an effect on CMV disease. It has to be given intravenously and is relatively non-toxic. Because of its chemical structure it may be deposited in bone but this has not produced problems in clinical use[122].

An obvious but important point to emphasize about CMV chemotherapy is that (as for other latent and persistent viruses) it is only active against replicating virus and cannot eradicate the virus from the host. The great importance of the host immune response in controlling CMV infection is illustrated by the accumulating experience with AIDS patients. Once these patients have had a major manifestation of CMV disease, relapse following the discontinuation of antiviral chemotherapy is extremely common. This is obviously not such a problem in clinical situations where there is an eventual likelihood of reversal of immunosuppression.

Interferon and cytosine arabinoside have also been used for the treatment of CMV but have been replaced by the antiviral agents discussed above. Hyperimmune globulin has been used but there is no convincing evidence of its efficacy.

Prophylaxis and vaccines

Perhaps the major aspect of prevention of CMV disease to emphasize is the importance of avoiding *primary* infection in seronegative immunosuppressed subjects by only giving them blood products and organs from seronegative donors. Hyperimmune globulin has also been used for the prophylaxis of CMV disease but (in the experience of the Seattle group) did not confer significant additional benefit over only giving seronegative blood products[123].

There is no vaccine of clearly established efficacy against CMV. The only candidate is an 'attenuated' Towne strain live CMV vaccine. However, there is no clearly defined marker for attenuation in human CMV (it cannot be tested in animals because it does not produce disease) and in trials this vaccine has not shown statistically significant prevention of acquisition of CMV in seronegative subjects, although it is claimed that vaccinees have less severe CMV disease when they become clinically infected[124]: infection with newly acquired CMV can be distinguished from reactivation of the vaccine strain by restriction endonuclease mapping of the isolates. In addition, there are strong theoretical reasons for preferring subunit (rather than live) vaccines for herpes viruses: CMV is a candidate oncogenic virus – obviously live vaccines could establish latency and whether this might present problems later is unknown.

Conclusion

It can be seen that much uncertainty still surrounds CMV. The slow growth of the virus in tissue culture, and the assumption that herpes simplex would serve as a paradigm for all herpes viruses, have resulted in relatively less attention being paid to the molecular virology of CMV. However, there is now increasing study of the virus at a molecular level, and this should result in a better understanding of the biology and pathogenesis of this somewhat enigmatic member of the herpes virus family.

VARICELLA ZOSTER AND HERPES SIMPLEX VIRUSES

This chapter has focussed on EBV and CMV, which have a particular propensity to produce problems in immunosuppressed patients.

VZV and HSV are both alpha herpes viruses whose site of persistence is within the nervous system – they both exhibit classical latency in neuronal cells within sensory ganglia. Although the incidence of disease related to VZV and HSV is appreciable in immunosuppressed patients, they are given less space in this review partly because there is little or no evidence they selectively infect cells of the immune system, and also because they are now relatively easily treated with appropriate antiviral therapy. However, the lesser space devoted to them here does not reflect any general lack of scientific attention. HSV is by far the most intensively studied herpes virus at a molecular level, and both it and VZV have now been completely sequenced[125].

Virology

Details of the molecular virology of HSV, and of the lesser body of knowledge on VZV, are available in recent reviews[126]. The viruses infect epithelial cells and then travel up axons to become latent in sensory ganglia. As neuronal cells are long lived, persistence of the viral genome could presumably be maintained without any virus replication. Periodically reactivation occurs and virus is transported down sensory axons and released where it infects, and replicates in, epithelial cells. The mechanism of latency and reactivation is the focus of much research, discussion of which is beyond the scope of this chapter. In brief the mechanism is unknown, but it is important to note that no viral proteins have been reproducibly detected during latency. However a recent report suggests that an 'anti-sense' RNA transcript from the region of the HSV genome encoding the first immediate early gene transcribed (known as ICP O), is present during latency. This would provide a mechanism for inhibiting transcription of 'sense' mRNA from this important gene, whose expression is a prerequisite for further viral gene transcription, and if verified will be of importance in understanding latency[127].

Epidemiology

Both VZV and HSV are ubiquitous with 80-90% of adults carrying both viruses, as determined by the presence of antibody. HSV 1 and 2 appear to be transmitted predominantly by direct contact, with oral or facial lesions for HSV1, and sexual contact for HSV2 which accounts for most genital herpes virus infections. VZV is transmitted by aerosol spread and direct contact. It is of course possible to acquire primary VZV infection (chicken pox) from a subject with zoster, whereas zoster is always a manifestation of reactivation.

Sites of persistence

In addition to their definite sites of latency in ganglia, VZV and HSV have also been reported to be present in lymphoid cells during acute active infection. VZV has been detected in peripheral blood lyphocytes of subjects with chickenpox and HSV has also been reported in lymphocytes. In addition, HSV has been shown to infect a proportion of peripheral blood lymphoid cells in vitro; and VZV has been reported to infect some B lymphoblastoid cell lines[128,129]. However there is no evidence to suggest that either virus persists or establishes latency in these cell lines in the normal host *in vivo*. HSV DNA sequences have also been reported in normal brain (outside of sensory ganglia) and whether the virus persists in a wider range of cells in the CNS is not really clear.

Immunology

VZV does not have an experimental model and will not infect the usual rodent models used by immunologists. However HSV readily produces infection in mice and the immunology of murine HSV infection has been extensively studied – although it must be remembered that it is not a natural infection of mice. It has been shown that following inoculation of virus into the ear pinna, T cells (Tc) mediating delayed hypersensitivity seem to play a major role in controlling infection – this has been shown by the classical techniques of depletion and adoptive transfer of Ly2$^+$3$^-$ cells. However HSV specific cytotoxic Tc also play a protective role, particularly following the i.v. injection of HSV – a less natural site of infection. Antibody may also play a role – the classical experiments of Stevens and Cooke in which HSV was first recovered from explanted mouse sensory ganglia, showed that recovery of virus by cocultivation was not possible if there was antibody to HSV in the medium[130]. More recently it has been interestingly shown that mice selectively depleted of B cells develop disseminated infection on challenge with HSV. The area has been well reviewed by Nash[131].

In humans it is supposed that effector T cell mediated immunity is of major importance in controlling persistent infection. This is inferred from the fact that reactivation and dissemination of virus occurs in the face of high titres of antibody, and that hypogammaglobulinaemic children do not experience severe HSV or VZV infection. In contrast severe disseminated HSV or VZV infection occurs in congenital T cell deficiency, and multidermatomal zoster is seen in patients with AIDS and in iatrogenically immunosuppressed patients.

The T cell response to HSV has been studied in humans, and it has been reported that HSV specific Tc can be generated from peripheral blood – however the reported Tc clones specific for HSV have all been class II restricted T4$^+$ cells – specificity of such clones for HSV glycoproteins has been reported but no systematic attempts to look for specificity for other viral proteins has been made[132]. Recently VZV specific Tc have also been generated from peripheral blood. Class II restricted VZV specific Tc clones have been described[133], and the frequency of class I restricted VZV specific Tc precursors has been estimated by limiting dilution analysis. This latter study showed that the frequency of VZV specific Tc in asymptomatic seropositive subjects was about 1 in 50000 or less – whereas these same authors found the frequency of CMV specific Tc was about 1 in 10–20000[134]. It may be that these different frequencies reflect the different sites of latency or persistence of alpha herpes viruses – although speculative it might be supposed that VZV, showing classical latency within neuronal cells, would not provide as much secondary *in vitro* restimulation as CMV or EBV which may maintain a low level of replication in the normal host. There is really no information on whether T cells specific for alpha herpes viruses show any specificity for non-structural proteins of HSV or VZV.

An important question about the role of immunity in alpha herpes virus infections is whether it plays any role in maintaining latency within neuronal cells, or only in limiting dissemination once reactivation and axonal spread to epithelial cells has occurred. In brief, there is no definite evidence for the immune response playing any role in maintaining latency and the immediate events involved in reactivation from latency seem more likely to be elucidated by understanding the molecular virology of HSV and VZV.

Clinical manifestations of VZV and HSV

The clinical syndrome of primary VZV infection – varicella (chicken pox) is well known and described in standard texts[135]. Vesicles occur predominantly on the trunk, but also on mucosal surfaces – these latter subsequently ulcerate and account for the spread of virus by the respiratory route. Varicella in immunosuppressed individuals can be an extremely severe and even fatal disease, characterized by dissemination to internal organs with pneumonitis being a particularly severe complication. Although X-ray evidence of pneumonia is not so uncommon in adults, there are rarely any clinical signs. However, severe varicella pneumonia is characterized by cough, dyspnoea, pleuritic pain and diffuse nodular shadowing on chest X-ray – the mortality was said to be around 10% (before the advent of acyclovir). Encephalitis and hepatitis are also features of dissemination, and haemorrhagic varicella with bleeding into vesicles may occur. Dissemination is commonest in children receiving chemotherapy or with absolute lymphopenia at the time of infection. Reactivation of VZV is characterized by the distribution of lesions within a sensory dermatome giving the well known picture of herpes zoster. This obviously results from reactivation and retrograde axonal spread from sensory ganglia. Infectious virus can be recovered from lesions until they become pustular and crust over. Reactivation of VZV in immunosuppressed individuals is again more severe than in normal subjects – blood borne dissemination occurs giving a clinical picture like varicella in addition to zoster. Patients with Hodgkin's disease seem particularly at risk of developing zoster (20–50% of patients), and multidermatomal zoster is now recognised to be a feature of AIDS.

Primary HSV infection is presumably often asymptomatic in the normal host, given the high incidence of seropositivity. Reactivation can produce the characteristic cold sores on the face, or in the genital area for HSV II. Why some otherwise normal individuals should be prone to recurrent episodes of reactivation of HSV, whilst most normal seropositive individuals are not is unknown. No consistent difference in the immune response to HSV has been shown in those who get recurrent reactivation[136]. The most serious clinical presentation of HSV is herpes simplex encephalitis – why this should occur in otherwise normal subjects is again unknown. There is no evidence that particular strains of HSV are neurovirulent, and in most cases encephalitis occurs in those already latently infected – presumably by reactivation from virus in the CNS or sensory ganglia. HSV infection in the immunosuppressed is again a common problem – herpes simplex stomatitis is common, and HSV oesophagitis, pneumonitis and hepatitis may occur. Reactivation, evidenced by virus shedding occurs in up to 80% of bone marrow transplant recipients. Recognition of HSV as the cause of these features in immunosuppressed individuals requires isolation of virus, or demonstration of virus by electron microscopy or immunoelectronmicroscopy. HSV has been suggested as an aetiological factor in other diseases on rather slender evidence. For instance it has been suggested that HSV may be involved in the pathogenesis of Behçet's disease as virus has been shown in the ulcers by hybridisation. The problem with such studies is that it is always possible that this just reflects secondary reactivation rather than any aetiological role. HSV has also been implicated in the causation of cervical cancer but its role is still controversial and much less certain than that of papilloma viruses. Further details on clinical aspects of VZV and HSV are available in recent reviews[137, 138].

Treatment

Both VZV and HSV can now be treated effectively with antiviral agents. Acyclovir (acycloguanosine) has now supplanted other antivirals previously used for treating HSV. It is a guanosine analogue which is phosphorylated to the monophosphate by the HSV or VZV specified thymidine kinase. It is then further phosphorylated to the triphosphate and incorporated into the new viral DNA strand. The virus DNA polymerase cannot read past the acyclovir triphosphate and chain elongation is blocked. Its specificity and lack of toxicity results from its only being phosphorylated to the active form in virus infected cells.

There is no doubt that it is highly effective in preventing HSV replication and in shortening the duration of reactivation episodes if given sufficiently early. It has also been shown to be effective in treating HSV encephalitis in multicentre trials. It is now used prophylactically by some centres in bone marrow transplant recipients.

Acyclovir is also effective in the treatment of VZV infection although prevention of viral replication *in vitro* requires higher concentrations than for HSV. It is recommended for treatment of VZV infection in the immunocompromised and should be given i.v. in a dose of 8mg/kg/day in divided doses. It has recently been recommended for the treatment of zoster in the *normal* host and claimed that treatment shortens the duration of the lesions and the acute pain. Topical acyclovir is also effective for herpes simplex keratitis[139].

There has been concern that the use of acyclovir would favour the emergence of thymidine kinase (TK) negative mutants, but although TK-virus can be isolated, this has not thus far proved a problem in practice. Indeed there is some evidence that TK-HSV is less effective in establishing latent infection. Of course acyclovir does not eradicate latent virus and is only effective when viral replication is occurring. Other agents which have been used to treat HSV and VZV such as vidarabine and interferons have now been supplanted by acyclovir. There is no evidence that isoprinosine (which has been promoted for the treatment of HSV) has any significant antiviral effect.

Prophylaxis and vaccines

There has been much interest in developing vaccines against HSV but there is no accepted or licensed vaccine in use at present. Claims have been made that a subunit vaccine made from the HSV glycoprotein D can prevent infection but this requires confirmation. Moss and colleagues, who have pioneered the use of recombinant vaccinia viruses as vectors for subunit vaccines, have shown that a vaccinia recombinant expressing HSV gD will protect mice from HSV infection[140]. It is generally agreed that a subunit vaccine is to be preferred. However in the case of VZV there is a *whole virus* vaccine available which seems likely to be licensed soon for use in humans – this is the 'Oka' vaccine and is a live attenuated strain of VZV. It has undergone trials in children with leukaemia or lymphoma and in nurses on wards caring for such patients. These suggest a protective effect of the vaccine[141]. The vaccine itself produces little or no symptoms, but as with all live vaccines derived from persistent viruses a crucial question is whether the vaccine strain persists. It appears that the Oka vaccine can establish persistence – as the implications for the host of an altered virus establishing persistence are uncertain, this is one of the main objections.

Passive immunization also has some role in the prevention of primary VZV infection. Varicella zoster immune globulin is indicated in those patients with immunodeficiency or malignancy, and those on steroids or cytotoxic therapy, who are susceptible and have known recent exposure to VZV. It is also indicated for neonates whose mothers develop varicella within 5 days of delivery[138].

References

1. Honess, R. W. (1984). Herpes simplex and 'the herpes complex': diverse observations and a unifying hypothesis. *J. Gen. Virol.*, **65**, 2077-107
2. Henle, G., Henle, W. and Diehl, V. (1968). Relation of Burkitt's tumour-associated herpes-types virus to infectious mononucleosis. *Proc. Natl. Acad. Sci, USA.*, **59**, 94-101
3. Epstein, M. A. (1978). Epstein-Barr virus-discovery, properties and relationship to nasopharyngeal carcinoma. In de-Thé, G., Ito, Y. and Davis, W. (eds.) *Nasopharyngeal Carcinoma: Aetiology and Control.* pp. 333-45. (Lyon: IARC)
4. Epstein, M. A. and Achong, B. G. (1979). The relationship of the virus to Burkitt's lymphoma. In Epstein, M. A. and Achong, B. G. (eds.) *The Epstein-Barr Virus.* pp. 321-337. (Berlin, Heidelberg, New York: Springer-Verlag)
5. Hanto, D. W., Frizzera, G., Gajl-Peczalska, K. J., Purtilo, D. T., Klein, G., Simmons, R. L. and Najarian, J. S. (1981). The Epstein-Barr virus (EBV) in the pathogenesis of post-transplant lymphoma. *Transplant. Proc.*, **13**, 756-60
6. Rickinson, A. B. (1986). Chronic, symptomatic Epstein-Barr virus infections. *Immunol. Today*, 7, 13-14
7. Purtilo, D. T., Cassel, C. K., Yang, J. P. S., Harper, R., Stevenson, S. R., Landing, B. H. and Vawter, G. F. (1975). X-linked recessive progressive combined variable immuno-deficiency (Duncan's disease). *Lancet*, **1**, 935-40
8. Crawford, D. H., Epstein, M. A., Achong, B. G., Finerty, S., Newman, J., Liversedge, S., Tedder, R. S. and Stewart, J. W. (1979). Virological and immunological studies on a fatal case of infectious mononucleosis. *J. Infect.*, **1**, 37-48
9. Baer, R., Bankier, A. T., Biggin, M. D., Deininger, P. L., Farrell, P. J., Gibson, T. J., Hatfull, G., Hudson, G. S., Satchwell, S. C., Séguin, C., Tuffnell, P. S. and Barrell, B. G. (1984). DNA sequence and expression of the B95-8 Epstein-Barr virus genome. *Nature (London)*, **310**, 207-11

10. Nemerow, G. R., Wolfert, R., McNaughton, M. E. and Cooper, N. R. (1985). Identification and characterisation of the EBV receptor on human B lymphocytes and its relationship to the C3d receptor (CR2). *J. Virol.*, **55**, 347–51

11. Nadler, L. M., Stashenko, P., Hardy, R., van Agthouen, A., Terhorst, C. and Schlossman, S. F. (1981). Characterisation of a human B cell specific antigen (B2) distinct from B1. *J. Immunol.*, **126**, 1941–3

12. Sixbey, J. W., Davis, D. S., Young, L. S., Hutt-Fletcher, L., Tedder, T. F. and Rickinson, A. B. (1987). *J. Gen. Virol.*, **68**, 805–11

13. Aman, P., Ehlin-Henriksson, B. and Klein, G. (1984). Epstein–Barr virus susceptibility to normal human B lymphocyte populations. *J. Exp. Med.*, **159**, 208–20

14. Tosato, G., Blaese, R. M. and Yarchoan, R. (1985). Relationship between immunoglobulin production and immortalisation by EB virus. *J. Immunol.*, **135**, 959–64

15. Rosen, A., Gergely, P., Jondal, M., Klein, G. and Britton, S. (1977). Polyclonal Ig production after Epstein–Barr virus infection of human lymphocytes *in vitro. Nature (London)*, **267**, 52–4

16. Azim, T. and Crawford, D. H. (1988). B lymphocyte differentiation and immortalisation are separate consequences of Epstein–Barr virus infection. *Int. J. Cancer*, (In press)

17. Pope, J. H., Horne, M. K. and Scott, W. (1968). Transformation of foetal human leucocytes *in vitro* by filtrates of a human leukaemia cell line containing herpes-like virus. *Int. J. Cancer*, **3**, 857–66

18. Thorley-Lawson, D. A., Nadler, L. M., Bhan, A. K. and Schooley, R. T. (1985). Blast-2 (EBVCS), an early cell surface marker of human B cell activation is superinduced by EBV. *J. Immunol.*, **134**, 3007–12

19. Thorley-Lawson, D. A. and Mann, K. P. (1985). Early events in Epstein–Barr virus infection provide a model for B cell activation. *J. Exp. Med.*, **162**, 45–9

20. Swenderman, S. and Thorley-Lawson, D. A. (1987). The activation antigen Blast-2, when shed, is an autocrine BCGF for normal and transformed B cells. *E.M.B.O. J.*, **6**, 1637–42

21. Blazer, B. A., Sutton, L. M. and Strome, M. (1983). Self-stimulating growth factor production by B-cell lines derived from Burkitt's lymphomas and other lines transformed *in vitro* by Epstein–Barr virus. *Cancer Res.*, **43**, 4562–8

22. Gordon, J., Ley, S. E., Melamed, M. D., English, L. S. and Hughes-Jones, N. C. (1984). Immortalised B lymphocytes produce B-cell growth factor. *Nature (London)*, **310**, 145–7

23. zur Hausen, H. and Henle, W. (1967). Comparative study of cultured Burkitt tumor cells by immunofluorescence, autoradiography and electron microscopy. *J. Virol.*, **1**, 830–7

24. Reedman, B. M. and Klein, G. (1973). Cellular localisation of an Epstein–Barr virus (EBV)-associated complement-fixing antigen in producer and non-producer lymphoblastoid cell lines. *Int. J. Cancer*, **11**, 499–520

25. Hennessy, K., Fennewald, S., Hummel, M., Cole, T. and Kieff, E. (1984). A membrane protein encoded by Epstein–Barr virus in latent growth transforming infection. *Proc. Natl. Acad. Sci, USA.*, **81**, 7207–11

26. Rawlins, D. R., Milman, G., Hayward, S. D. and Hayward, G. S. (1985). Sequence-specific DNA binding of the Epstein–Barr virus nuclear antigen (EBNA-1) to clustered sites in the plasmid maintenance region. *Cell*, **42**, 859–68

27. Wang, D., Liebowitz, D. and Klieff, E. (1985). An EBV membrane protein expressed in immortalised lymphocytes transforms established rodent cells. *Cell*, **43**, 831–40

28. Rowe, D. T., Rowe, M., Evans, G. I., Wallace, L. E., Farrell, P. J. and Rickinson, A. B. (1986). Restricted expression of EBV latent genes and T-lymphocyte-detected membrane antigen in Burkitt's lymphoma cells. *E.M.B.O. J.*, **5**, 2599–608

29. Sixbey, J. W., Vestemien, E. H., Nedrud, J. G., Raab-Traub, N., Walton, L. A. and Pagano, J. S. (1983). Replication of Epstein–Barr virus in human epithelial cells infected *in vitro. Nature (London)*, **306**, 480–3

30. Sixbey, J. W., Nedrud, J. G., Raab-Traub, N., Hanes, R. A. and Pagano, J. S. (1984). Epstein–Barr virus replication in oropharyngeal epithelial cells. *N. Engl. J. Med.*, **310**, 1225–30

31. Sixbey, J. W., Lemon, S. M. and Pagano, J. S. (1986). A second site for Epstein–Barr virus shedding: the uterine cervix. *Lancet*, **2**, 1122–4

32. Wolf, H., zur Hausen, H. and Becker, V. (1973). EB viral genomes in epithelial nasopharyngeal carcinoma cells. *Nat. New Biol.*, **244**, 245

33. Taichman, L. B., Reilly, S. S. and La Porta, R. F. (1983). The role of keratinocyte differentiation in the expression of epitheliotropic viruses. *J. Invest. Dermatol.*, **81**, 137s–40s

34. Crawford, D. H. and Ando, I. (1986). EB virus induction is associated with B cell maturation. *Immunology*, **59**, 405–9

35. Hewetson, J. F., Rocchi, G., Henle, W. and Henle, G. (1973). Neutralising antibodies to Epstein–Barr virus in healthy populations and patients with infectious mononucleosis. *J. Infect. Dis.*, **128**, 283–9

36. Evans, A. S., Niederman, J. C. and McCollum, R. W. (1968). Seroepidemiologic studies of infectious mononucleosis with EB virus. *N. Engl. J. Med.*, **279**, 1121–7

37. Golden, H. D., Chang, R. S., Prescott, W., Simpson, E. and Cooper, T. Y. (1973). Leukocyte-transforming agent: prolonged excretion by patients with mononucleosis and excretion by normal individuals. *J. Infect. Dis.*, **127**, 471–3

38. Klein, G., Swedmyr, E., Jondal, U. and Persson, P. O. (1976). EBV-determined nuclear antigens (EBNA)-positive cells in the peripheral blood of infectious mononucleosis patients. *Int. J. Cancer*, **17**, 21–6

39. Rhodes, G., Carson, D. A., Valbracht, J., Houghten, R. and Vaughan, J. H. (1985). Human immune responses to synthetic peptides from the Epstein–Barr nuclear antigen. *J. Immunol.*, **134**, 211–16

40. Henle, W., Henle, G., Andersson, J., Ernberg, I., Klein, G., Horwitz, C. A., Marklund, G., Rymo, L., Wellinder, C. and Straus, S. E. (1987). Antibody responses to Epstein–Barr virus-determined nuclear antigen (EBNA)-1 and EBNA-2 in acute and chronic Epstein–Barr virus infection. *Proc. Natl. Acad. Sci. USA.*, **84**, 570–4

41. Crawford, D. H., Brickell, P., Tidman, N., McConnell, I., Hoffbrand, A. V. and Janossy, J. (1981). Increased numbers of cells with suppressor T cell phenotype in the peripheral blood of patients with infectious mononucleosis. *Clin. Exp. Immunol.*, **43**, 291–7

42. Rickinson, A. B., Moss, D. J., Pope, J. H. and Ahlberg, N. (1980). Long-term T-cell-mediated immunity to Epstein–Barr virus in man. IV. Development of T-cell memory in convalescent infectious mononucleosis patients. *Int. J. Cancer*, **25**, 59–65

43. Tosato, G., Magrath, I., Koski, I., Dooley, N. and Blaese, M. (1979). Activation of suppressor T cells during Epstein–Barr-virus-induced infectious mononucleosis. *N. Engl. J. Med.*, **301**, 1133–7

44. Rickinson, A. B., Strang, G., Murray, R. and Rowe, M. (1987). Cellular controls over to EB virus infection. Levine, P. H. (ed.) Proceedings of the *2nd International Symposium on EBV and related diseases*. (Clifton, New Jersey: Humana Press)

45. Nilsson, K., Klein, G., Henle, W. and Henle, G. (1971). The establishment of lymphoblastoid lines from adult and foetal human lymphoid cells and its dependence on EBV. *Int. J. Cancer*, **8**, 443–50

46. Pearson, G. R. and Orr, T. W. (1976). Antibody-dependent lymphocyte cytotoxicity against cells expressing Epstein–Barr virus antigens. *J. Natl. Cancer Inst.*, **56**, 485–8

47. Moss, D. J., Rickinson, A. B. and Pope, J. H. (1978). Long-term T-cell-mediated immunity to Epstein–Barr virus in man. I. Complete regression of virus-induced transformation in cultures of seropositive donor leucocytes. *Int. J. Cancer*, **22**, 662–8

48. Henle, W. and Henle, G. (1981). Epstein–Barr virus-specific serology in immunologically compromised individuals. *Cancer Res.*, **41**, 4222–5

49. Crawford, D. H., Edwards, J. M. B., Sweny, P., Hoffbrand, A. V. and Janossy, G. (1981). Studies on long-term T-cell-mediated immunity to Epstein–Barr virus in immuno-suppressed renal allograft recipients. *Int. J. Cancer*, **28**, 705–9

50. Penn, I. (1979). Tumour incidence in human allograft recipients. *Transplant. Proc.*, **11**, 1047–51

51. Crawford, D. H., Thomas, J. A., Janossy, G., Sweny, P., Fernando, O. N., Moorhead, J. F. and Thompson, J. H. (1980). Epstein–Barr virus nuclear antigen positive lymphoma after cyclosporin A treatment in patient with renal allograft. *Lancet*, **1**, 1355–60

52. Hanto, D. W., Frizzera, G., Purtilo, D. T., Sakamoto, K., Sullivan, J., Saemundsen, A. K., Klein, G., Simmons, R. L. and Najarian, J. S. (1981). Clinical spectrum of lymphoproliferative disorders in renal transplant recipients and evidence for the role of Epstein–Barr virus. *Cancer Res.*, **41**, 4253–61

53. Cleary, M. L., Dorfman, R. F. and Sklar, J. (1986). Failure in immunological control of

the virus infection: post-transplant lymphomas. In Epstein, M. A. and Achong, B. G. (eds.) *The Epstein–Barr Virus Recent Advances.* pp. 163–82. (London: William Heinemann)

54. Hanto, D. W., Frizzera, G., Gajl-Peczalska, K. J., Sakamoto, K., Purtilo, D. T., Balfour, H. H., Simmons, R. L. and Najarian, J. S. (1982). Acyclovir therapy and transition from polyclonal to monoclonal B-cell proliferation. *N. Engl. J. Med.*, **306**, 913–18

55. Collins, P. (1983). The spectrum of antiviral activities of acyclovir *in vitro* and *in vivo*. *J. Antimicrobial Chemotherapy*, **12**, suppl. B, 19–27

56. Purtilo, D. T., de Florio, D., Hutt, L. M., Bhawan, J., Yang, J. P. S., Otto, R. and Edwards, W. (1977). Variable phenotypic expression of an X-linked recessive lymphoproliferative syndrome. *N. Engl. J. Med.*, **297**, 1077–81

57. Purtilo, D. T. (1983). Immunopathology of X-linked lymphoproliferative syndrome. *Immunol. Today*, **4**, 291–6

58. Ando, I., Morgan, G., Levinsky, R. J. and Crawford, D. H. (1986). A family of the X-linked lymphoproliferative syndrome: evidence for a B cell defect contributing to the immunodeficiency. *Clin. Exp. Immunol.*, **63**, 271–9

59. Tosato, G., Straus, S., Henle, W., Pike, S. E. and Blaese, B. M. (1985). Characteristic T cell dysfunction in patients with chronic active Epstein–Barr virus infection (chronic infectious mononucleosis). *J. Immunol.*, **134**, 3082–8

60. Schooley, R. T., Carey, R. W., Miller, G., Henle, W., Eastman, R., Mark, E. J., Kenyon, K., Wheeler, E. O. and Rubin, R. H. (1986). Chronic Epstein–Barr virus infection associated with fever and interstitial pneumonitis. *Ann. Intern. Med.*, **104**, 636–43

61. Horwitz, C., Henle, W., Henle, G. and Schmitz, H. (1975). Clinical evaluation of patients with infectious mononucleosis and development of antibodies to the R component of the Epstein–Barr virus-induced early antigen complex. *Am. J. Med.*, **58**, 330–8

62. Jones, J. F., Ray, G., Minnich, L. L., Hicks, M. J., Ribler, R. and Lucas, D. O. (1985). Evidence of active Epstein–Barr virus infection in patients with persistent unexplained illness: elevated anti-early antigen antibodies. *Ann. Intern. Med.*, **102**, 1–7

63. Borysiewicz, L. K., Haworth, S. J., Cohen, J., Mundin, J., Rickinson, A. and Sissons, G. P. (1986). Epstein–Barr virus-specific immune defects in patients with persistent symptoms following infectious mononucleosis. *Q. J. Med.*, **58**, 226, 111–21

64. Burkitt, D. (1958). A sarcoma involving the jaws in African children. *Br. J. Surg.*, **46**, 218–23

65. Epstein, M. A., Barr, Y. M. and Achong, B. G. (1964). Virus particles in cultured lymphoblasts from Burkitt's lymphoma. *Lancet*, **1**, 702–3

66. Zimler, U., Addinger, H. K., Lenoir, G. M., Uuillaume, M., Knebel-Doeberitz, M. V., Laux, G., Désgranges, C., Wittmann, P., Freese, V-K., Schneider, U. and Bornkamm, G. W. (1986). Geographical prevalence of two types of Epstein–Barr virus. *Virology*, **154**, 55–6

67. Ernberg, I., Kallin, B., Dillner, J., Falk, K., Ehlin-Henriksson, B., Hammarskiold, M-L. and Klein, G. (1986). Lymphoblastoid cell lines and Burkitt lymphoma-derived cell lines differ in the expression of a second Epstein–Barr virus encoded nuclear antigen. *Int. J. Cancer*, **38**, 729–37

68. de-Thé, G. (1979). Demographic studies implicating the virus in the causation of Burkitt's lymphoma; prospects for nasopharyngeal carcinoma. In Epstein, M. A. and Achong, B. G. (eds.) *The Epstein–Barr Virus.* pp. 417–35. (Berlin, Heidelberg, New York: Springer-Verlag)

69. Pope, J. H., Scott, W. and Moss, D. J. (1974). Cell relationships in transformation of human leucocytes by Epstein– Barr virus. *Int. J. Cancer*, **14**, 122–9

70. Shope, T., Dechaero, D. and Miller, G. (1973). Malignant lymphoma in cotton top marmosets after inoculation with Epstein–Barr virus. *Proc. Natl. Acad. Sci. USA.*, **70**, 2487–91

71. Whittle, H., Brown, J., Marsh, K., Greenwood, B. M., Seidelin, P., Tighe, H. and Wedderburn, L. (1984). T-cell control of Epstein–Barr virus-infected B cells is lost during *P. falciparum* malaria. *Nature*, **312**, 449–50

72. Manolov, G. and Manolova, Y. (1972). Marker band in one chromosome 14 from Burkitt lymphomas. *Nature (London)*, **237**, 33–4

73. Klein, G. and Klein, E. (1985). Myc/Ig juxtaposition by chromosomal translocations: some new insights, puzzles and paradoxes. *Immunol. Today*, **6**, 208–15

74. Haluska, F. G., Tsujimoto, T. and Croce, C. M. (1987). Mechanisms of chromosome translocation in B- and T-cell neoplasia. *Trends in Genetics*, 2, 11-15
75. Rooney, C. M., Rowe, M., Wallace, L. E. and Rickinson, A. B. (1985). Epstein-Barr virus-positive Burkitt's lymphoma cells not recognised by virus-specific T-cell surveillance. *Nature (London)*, 317, 629-31
76. Ito, Y. (1986). Vegetable activators of the viral genome and the causation of Burkitt's lymphoma and nasopharyngeal carcinoma. In Epstein, M. A. and Achong, B. G. (eds.) *The Epstein-Barr Virus Recent Advances*. pp. 207-36. (London: William Heinemann)
77. Crawford, D. H., Epstein, M. A., Bornkamm, G. W., Achong, B. G., Finerty, S. and Thompson, J. L. (1979). Biological and biochemical observations on isolates of EB virus from the malignant epithelial cells of two nasopharyngeal carcinomas. *Int. J. Cancer*, 24, 294-302
78. Epstein, M. A. (1986). Vaccination against Epstein-Barr virus: current progress and future strategies. *Lancet*, 1, 1425-7
79. Epstein, M. A., Morgan, A. J., Finerty, S., Randle, B. J. and Kirkwood, J. K. (1985). Protection of cotton top tamarins against Epstein-Barr virus-induced malignant lymphoma by a prototype subunit vaccine. *Nature (London)*, 318, 287-9
80. Epstein, M. A., Randle, B. J., Finerty, S. and Kirkwood, J. K. (1986). Not all potently neutralising vaccine-induced antibodies to Epstein-Barr virus ensure protection of susceptible experimental animals. *Clin. Exp. Immunol.*, 63, 485-90
81. Old, L. J., Boyse, E. A., Oettgen, H. F., de Harven, E., Geering, G., Williamson, B. and Clifford, P. (1966). Precipitated antibody in human serum to an antigen present in cultured Burkitt's lymphoma cells. *Proc. Natl. Acad. Sci. USA*, 56, 1699-704
82. Tobi, M. and Straus, E. (1985). Chronic Epstein-Barr virus disease: a workshop held by the National Institute of Allergy and Infectious Diseases. *Ann. Intern. Med.*, 103, 951-3
83. Akaboshi, I., Katsuki, T., Jamamoto, J. and Matsuda, I. (1983). Unique pattern of Epstein-Barr virus specific antibodies in recurrent parotitis. *Lancet*, 2, 1049-51
84. Andiman, W. A., Eastman, R., Martin, K., Katz, B. Z., Rubinstein, A., Pitt, J., Pahwa, S. and Miller, G. (1985). Opportunistic lymphoproliferations associated with Epstein-Barr viral DNA in infants and children with AIDS. *Lancet*, 2, 1390-3
85. Vergnon, J. M., Vincent, M., de Thé, G., Momex, J. F., Weynants, P. and Boune, J. (1984). Cryptogenic fibrosing alveolitis and Epstein-Barr virus: an association? *Lancet*, 2, 768-71
86. Greenspan, J. S., Greenspan, D., Lenette, E. T., Abrams, D. I., Conant, M. A., Petersen, V. and Freese, U.K. (1985). Replication of Epstein-Barr virus within the epithelial cells of oral 'hairy' leukoplakia, an AIDS-associated lesion. *N. Engl. J. Med.*, 313, 1564-71
87. Hayward, G. S. (1986). Herpes viruses – genome structure and regulations. In *Cancer Cells*, Vol. 4: DNA tumour viruses.
88. Stenberg, R. M., Wittle, P. R. and Stinski, M. F. (1985). Multiple spliced and unspliced transcripts from human CMV immediate early region 2, and evidence for a common initiation site within immediate early region 1. *J. Virol.*, 56, 665-75
89. Crannage, M. P., Kouzarides, T., Bankier, A. T. *et al.* (1986). Identification of the human CMV glycoprotein B gene and induction of neutralising antibodies via its expression in recombinant vaccinia virus. *EMBO J.*, 5, 3057
90. Gonczol, E., Andrews, P. W. and Plotkin, S. A. (1984). CMV replicates in differentiated but not in undifferentiated human embryonal carcinoma cells. *Science*, 224, 159-61
91. Schrier, R., Nelson, J. A. and Oldstone, M. B. A. (1985). Detection of human CMV in peripheral blood lymphocytes in a natural infection. *Science*, 230, 1048-50
92. Jordan, C. *et al.* (1987). Neutrophils as a site of CMV persistence. *Fed. Proc.*
93. Rice, G. P., Schrier, R. D. and Oldstone, M. B. A. (1984). CMV infection of human lymphocytes and monocytes: virus expression is restricted to immediate early gene products. *Proc. Natl. Acad. Sci. USA*, 81, 6134-8
94. Einhorn, L. and Ost, A. (1984). CMV infection of human blood cells. *J. Infect. Dis.*, 149, 207-14
95. Rubin, R. H., Cosimi, A. B., Tolkoff-Rubin, N. E. *et al.* (1977). Infectious disease syndromes attributable to CMV and their significance among renal transplant recipients. *Transplantation*, 24, 458-64
96. Rinaldo, C. R. and Hirsch, M. S. (1980). Mechanisms of immunosuppression in cytomegaloviral mononucleosis. *J. Infect. Dis.*, 141, 488-95

97. Carney, W. P. and Hirsch, M. S. (1981). Mechanisms of immunosuppression in CMV mononucleosis. II. Virus monocyte interactions. *J. Infect. Dis.*, **144**, 47–54
98. Rodgers, B. C., Scott, D. M., Mundin, J. C. and Sissons, J. G. P. (1985). Monocyte derived inhibitor of interleukin 1 induced by human cytomegalovirus. *J. Virol.*, **55**, 527–32
99. Schrier, R. D., Rice, G. P. A. and Oldstone, M. B. A. (1986). Suppression of natural killer cell activity and T cell proliferation by fresh isolates of human cytomegalovirus. *J. Infect. Dis.*, **153**, 1084–91
100. Borysiewicz, L. K., Morris, S. M., Page, J. and Sissons, J. G. P. (1983). Human CMV specific cytotoxic T lymphocytes: requirements for *in vitro* generation and specificity. *Eur. J. Immunol.*, **13**, 804–9
101. Borysiewicz, L. K., Graham, S., Hickling, J. K. and Sissons, J. G. P. (1988). Human CMV specific cytotoxic T lymphocytes: limiting dilution analysis of cytotoxic T cells directed to late and early viral antigens (in press)
102. Townsend, A. R. M., Rothbard, J., Gotch, F. M. *et al.* (1986). The epitopes of influenza nucleoprotein recognised by cytotoxic T lymphocytes can be defined with short synthetic peptides. *Cell*, **44**, 959–68
103. Reddehase, M. S., Keil, G. M. and Koszinowski, U. H. (1984). The cytolytic T lymphocyte response to the murine cytomegalovirus. II. Detection of virus replication stage-specific antigens by separate populations of *in vivo* activated cytolytic T lymphocyte precursors. *Eur. J. Immunol.*, **14**, 56–61
104. Reddehase, M. J., Matter, W., Munch, K. *et al.* (1988). CD8⁺ T lymphocytes specific for murine CMV immediate early antigens mediate protective immunity. *J. Virol.*, (in press)
105. Borysiewicz, L. K., Rodgers, B., Morris, S., Graham, S. and Sissons, J. G. P. (1985). Lysis of human CMV infected fibroblasts by NK cells: demonstration of an interferon-independent component requiring expression of early viral proteins and characterization of effector cells. *J. Immunol.*, **134**, 2695–701
106. Bukowski, J. F., Warner, J. F., Dennert, G. *et al.* (1985). Adoptive transfer studies demonstrating the antiviral effect of natural killer cells *in vivo*. *J. Exp. Med.*, **161**, 40–52
107. Quinnan, G. V., Kimani, N., Esber, E. *et al.* (1981). HLA restricted cytotoxic T lymphocyte and nonthymic cytotoxic lymphocyte responses to CMV infection of bone marrow transplant recipients. *J. Immunol.*, **126**, 2036–41
108. Rook, A. H., Masur, H., Lane, H. C. *et al.* (1983). Interleukin-2 enhances the depressed natural killer and cytomegalovirus-specific cytotoxic activities of lymphocytes from patients with acquired immune deficiency syndrome. *J. Clin. Invest.*, **72**, 398–403
109. Ho, M. (1985). Cytomegalovirus. In Mandell G. *et al.* (ed.) *Principles and Practice of Infectious Disease*. pp. 960–970. (New York: John Wiley)
110. Griffiths, P. D., Stirk, P. R., Ganczakowski, M. *et al.* (1984). Rapid diagnosis of CMV infection in immunocompromised patients by detection of early antigen fluorescent foci. *Lancet*, **2**, 1242–4
111. Meyers, J. D., Flournoy, M. and Thomas, E. D (1986). Risk factors for CMV infection after human marrow transplantation. *J. Infect. Dis.*, **153**, 478–88
112. Glenn, J. (1981). CMV infections following renal transplantation. *Rev. Infect. Dis.*, **3**, 1151–77
113. Myerson, D., Hackman, R. C., Nelson, S. A. *et al.* (1983). *Human Pathol.*, **15**, 430–9
114. Barnes, D. M. (1987). Brain damage by AIDS under active study. *Science*, **235**, 1574–7
115. Schooley, R. T., Hirsch, M. S., Colvin, R. B. *et al.* (1983). Association of herpesvirus infections with T-lymphocyte subset alterations, glomerulopathy and opportunistic infections after renal transplantation. *N. Engl. J. Med.*, **308**, 307–13
116. Richardson, W. P., Colvin, R. B., Cheeseman, S. H. *et al.* (1981). Glomerulopathy associated with CMV viraemia in renal allografts. *N. Engl. J. Med.*, **305**, 57–63
117. Grundy, J. E., Shanley, J. D. and Shearer, G. M. (1985). Augmentation of graft-versus-host reaction by cytomegalovirus infection resulting in interstitial pneumonitis. *Transplantation*, **39**, 548–53
118. Stagno, S., Pass, R. F., Dworsky, M. E. *et al.* (1982). Congenital CMV infection – the relative importance of primary and recurrent maternal infection. *N. Engl. J. Med.*, **306**, 945–9
119. Preece, P. M., Pearl, K. N. and Peckham, C. S. (1984). Congenital CMV infection. *Arch. Dis. Child.*, **59**, 1120–6

120. Spector, D. H. and Spector, S. A. (1984). The oncogenic potential of human CMV. *Prog. Med. Virol.*, **29**, 45–89

121. Report of DHPG Study Group (1986). Treatment of serious cytomegalovirus infections with 9-(1, 3-dihydroxy-2-propoxymethyl) guanine in patients with AIDS and other immunodeficiencies. *N. Engl. J. Med.*, **314**, 801

122. Klintmalm, G., Lonnquist, B., Oberg, B. *et al.* (1985). Intravenous foscarnet for the treatment of severe CMV infection in allograft recipients. *Scand. J. Infect. Dis.*, **17**, 157–63

123. Bowden, R. A., Sayers, M., Flournoy, M. *et al.* (1986). CMV immune globulin and seronegative blood products to prevent primary CMV infection after marrow transplantation. *N. Engl. J. Med.*, **314**, 1006–19

124. Plotkin, S. A., Friedman, H. M., Fleisher, G. R. *et al.* (1984). Towne-vaccine-induced prevention of cytomegalovirus disease after renal transplants. *Lancet*, **1**, 528–31

125. Davison, A. J. and Scott, J. E. (1987). Complete DNA sequence of VZV. *J. Gen. Virol.*, **67**, 1759–816

126. Roizman, B. and Batterson, W. (1985). Herpes viruses and their replication. In Fields, B. N. *et al.* (eds) *Virology.* pp. 607–636. (New York: Raven Press)

127. Stevens, J. G., Wagner, E. K., Devi Rao, G. *et al.* (1987). RNA complementary to a herpes virus alpha gene is prominent in latently infected neurones. *Science*, **235**, 1056–8

128. Braun, P. W., Teute, H. K., Kirchner, H. *et al.* (1984). Replication of HSV in T lymphocytes. *J. Immunol.*, **132**, 914–19

129. Gilden, D. G. *et al.* (1987). Varicella zoster virus in mononuclear cells. *Virus Res.*, **7**, 117–29

130. Stevens, J. G. and Cooke, M. L. (1974). Mechanism of latent herpetic infection - an apparent role for anti-viral IgG. *J. Immunol.*, **113**, 1685–93

131. Nash, A. A. *et al.* (1986). The T cell mediated immune response of mice to herpes simplex virus. In Roismann, B. (ed.) *The Herpes Viruses.* Vol. 4, p. 87

132. Yasukawa, M. and Zarling, J. M. (1985). Human cytotoxic T cell clones against herpes simplex virus infected cells. *J. Immunol.*, **134**, 2679–82

133. Hayward, A. R., Pontesilli, O., Herberger, M. *et al.* (1986). Specific lysis of VZV infected B lymphoblasts by human T cells. *J. Virol.*, **58**, 179–84

134. Hickling, J. K., Borysiewicx, L. K. and Sissons, J. G. P. (1987). Varicella zoster virus specific cytotoxic T lymphocytes (Tc): detection and frequency analysis of HLA Class I restricted Tc in human peripheral blood. *J. Virol.*, **61**, 3463–9

135. Gelb, L. D. (1985). Varicella zoster virus. In Fields, B. N. (ed.) *Virology.* pp. 561–627. (New York: Raven Press)

136. Reviewed in Rawls, W. E. (1985). Herpes simplex virus. In Fields, B. N. (ed.) *Virology.* pp. 527–561. (New York: Raven Press)

137. Weller, T. H. (1983). Varicella herpes zoster virus - changing concepts of natural history control and importance of a not so benign virus. *N. Engl. J. Med.*, **309**, 1362–8

138. Brunell, P. A. (1985). Varicella zoster virus. In Mandell, G. L. *et al.* (eds.) *Principles and Practice of Infectious Disease.* pp. 952–960. (New York: Wiley Medical)

139. Shepp, D. H., Dandliker, P. S. and Meyers, J. D. (1986). Treatment of VZV infections in severely immunocompromised patients - a randomised comparison of acyclovir and vidaribine. *N. Engl. J. Med.*, **314**, 208–12

140. Cremer, K. J., Mackett, M., Wohlenberg, C. *et al.* (1985). Vaccinia virus recombinant expressing the HSV type-1 glycoprotein D prevents latent herpes in mice. *Science*, **228**, 737–9

141. Gershon, A. A. (1985). Live attenuted varicella vaccine. *J. Inf. Dis.*, **152**, 859–62

5
Clinical Significance of IgG Subclass and IgA Deficiency

L. Å. HANSON, J. BJÖRKANDER, R. SÖDERSTRÖM AND T. SÖDERSTRÖM

HISTORICAL ASPECTS

Hypogammaglobulinaemia was first described in a patient with severe infections by Bruton in 1952[1], and selective lack of IgA was initially noted in healthy individuals by Rockey et al. in 1964[2]. Lack of both serum and secretory IgA was later found to be the most common immunodeficiency. It occurs with a frequency from one in 396 to one in 886 (mean 1/568) in various normal healthy populations such as blood donors, of which altogether 394 629 have been tested[3]. IgA deficiency is more prevalent among patients with frequent infections, allergy or cancer[3-5].

IgG subclass deficiency was first noted by Terry in 1968[6] in patients with frequent infections. His study was followed by several reports[7-11]. Clearly such patients are common, and probably represent the most common immunodeficiency, although at the present time there are no reliable prevalence data[12].

Combined deficiencies of IgA and IgG subclasses were described a few years ago. These patients appear to be prone to respiratory infections, as first indicated by Oxelius et al.[13], and then supported by subsequent studies[14, 15]. However, in one large group of children with IgA deficiency, IgG subclass deficiency did not increase the risk of infection[16]. The reason for this discrepancy is not obvious, but could be due to the transient nature of the subclass deficiency in some children. Lowered levels of IgG subclasses are also seen in patients with other immunodeficiencies such as ataxia-telangiectasia[7, 17, 18]. IgA deficient individuals with high titres of anti-IgA may constitute a separate group where IgG4 and IgE are also low[19].

GENETICS OF IgA AND IgG SUBCLASS DEFICIENCIES

IgA deficiency

This is usually sporadic, but many family cases have been reported as recently reviewed[3]. Several investigators have searched for a connection between this deficiency and HLA haplotypes with differing conclusions, although a relation to HLA-A1/B8 was found, especially if the patients also had autoimmune disease[20-22]. More recently, Hammarström et al. found an increased frequency of HLA-B8/DR3 in healthy IgA deficient individuals, whereas B40 was significantly increased in those with IgA deficiency and frequent infections when compared to normals[23].

Various chromosomal abnormalities have been noted in patients with IgA deficiency, especially on chromosome 18. They have mostly had other unusual clinical features; the chromosomal abnormalities have also occurred without concurrent IgA deficiency[24-27].

No structural Cα-gene deletions were found among 85 blood donors with IgA deficiency[28]. With a hybridization-in-solution technique the same authors noted that α-chain mRNA was undetectable in polyclonally activated lymphocytes from individuals without detectable IgA[29].

IgG subclass deficiencies

These can be seen in families of patients with other immunodeficiencies. Thus IgG3 deficiency was noted in relatives of patients with common variable immunodeficiency and IgA deficiency, but also in other diseases such as diabetes mellitus type 1, SLE and C2 deficiency, the latter being due to a defect on chromosome 6[30]. These findings suggest an association between abnormalities of gene products on chromosomes 6 and 14, the latter carrying the Ig heavy chain genes.

Low levels of IgG3 are associated with the G3m(g) phenotype[31,32]. There is a strong linkage disequilibrium between the Glm(a) and G3m(g) genes and in IgG3 deficient patients Glm(+a) is found in increased frequency[33]. Those homozygous for G3m(g) had lower serum IgG3 levels than those who were heterozygous.

Gene deletions have been defined in a few cases of IgG subclass deficiencies[34,35]. Most patients with lowered levels of one or more subclasses probably have regulatory abnormalities.

CHANGING PATTERNS WITH AGE

IgA deficiency

Savilathi and Pelkonen[36] and Østergaard[37] have noted that IgA deficiency can be transient in children. However, severe IgA deficiency ($<$0.05 g/l in serum and secretory IgA undetectable) is permanent[38]. In a recent study by Plebani et al.[39], this was clearly illustrated by comparing children with severe deficiency to those with serum IgA levels $>$0.05 g/l, but below –2SD for age. The deficiency was permanent for the low group, but half of those with partial deficiency reached normal levels at a median time of 4 years after diagnosis, at a median age of 14 years. Gillon et al. noted that four out of 12 IgA deficient blood donors normalized their IgA levels within 6 months[40]. However, their initial serum levels were from 0.30 to 0.48 g/l. Finally, IgA deficiency secondary to exposure to drugs such as penicillamine, gold and phenytoins usually reverts to normal after the drug is discontinued[3].

IgG subclass deficiency

This is about three times more common in boys than girls, but the sex ratio reverses after puberty so that it is three times as common in women as men. In parallel there is a switch from a dominance of IgG2 deficiency in children to a predominance of IgG3 deficiency in adults[41, 42]. Transiently low levels of IgG subclasses have been noted in some children[16]. Variability of IgG subclass levels over time have been reported in children with chronic rhinosinusitis, otitis media and in some cases of pneumonia[43].

It should be noted that IgG2 and IgG4 production is relatively delayed during the normal ontogeny of the immune response in young children[44]. Before the age of 2 years children may respond poorly to polysaccharide antigens which primarily induce IgG2 antibodies. IgG1 antibodies are often produced instead, although it has been suggested that they may be of lower avidity than the IgG2 antibodies, and therefore possibly less protective[45].

Three cases are described with isolated IgG subclass deficiencies which progressed to a deficiency of all subclasses and a low total IgG[46]. One of these patients then reversed to isolated IgG3 deficiency. The regulatory abnormalities behind such fluctuations are unkown. In an *in vitro* study in five patients, Quinti *et al.*[47] showed that most had a B cell defect, sometimes associated with decreased T helper cell or increased T suppressor activity.

DISTRIBUTION OF ANTIBODIES IN IgA AND IN IgG ISOTYPES

The clinical relevance of IgA deficiency may be related to a lack of secretory IgA antibodies which are of major importance for protection of mucous membranes, where most infections are initiated[48]. There is little evidence that serum IgA antibodies participate in host defence, in fact Griffiss *et al.* have shown that serum IgA antibodies to meningococci may block the protective bactericidal activity to these bacteria[49]. On the other hand, there is a wealth of information that secretory IgA antibodies found in exocrine secretions, and on all mucous membranes, participate in defence against viruses and bacteria. They may do so primarily by binding to the microorgansims and preventing them from attaching to the mucosa which is usually the first step in the infectious process[48]. Antibodies of the secretory IgA class against a variety of microbes and food proteins, which come into contact with mucous membranes, are present in most secretions[48]. The subclass of IgG specific antibodies differ for various antigens, that is IgG antibodies against proteins are mainly IgG1 and IgG3, whereas antibodies to polysaccharides are mainly IgG2. The regulatory background to this division is unknown. Yount *et al.*[50] showed that antibodies against the polysaccharides levan, dextran and teichoic acid were primarily IgG2. This is also true of antibodies to phosphorylcholine and the C type polysaccharide cell wall antigen of pneumococci, group O and H streptococci, lactobacilli, nematodes and some fungi. In contrast IgG antibodies to proteins such as tetanus toxoid and most viral antigens are mainly IgG1 or IgG3. Mothers having the rare blood group p, who are prone to early spontaneous abortion or still birth, have antibodies against the p antigen which are almost exclusively IgG3[51]. Antibodies to viruses such as CMV, varicella, herpes zoster, herpes simplex and mumps are usually IgG1 and/or IgG3[52,53]. Linde[54] demonstrated IgG1 and IgG3 antibodies against rubella virus, although in 97 samples she found a few with IgG4 and one with IgG2 antibodies. Antibodies to food proteins are mainly IgG1[55].

IgG4 has been proposed as a possible reaginic antibody[56,57], but this has been questioned[58]. IgG4 may even act as a blocking antibody[59-61].

CLINICAL SIGNIFICANCE OF IgA DEFICIENCY

Lack of IgA in serum and secretions was the first immunodeficiency to be found in healthy individuals[2]. On the other hand, IgA deficiency is also associated with a number of conditions such as atopy, malignancies in the gastro-intestinal tract and the lymphoreticular system and malabsorption, including coeliac disease. Furthermore, autoimmune diseases such as idiopathic thrombocytopenic purpura, haemolytic anaemia, thyroiditis, dermatomyositis, chronic active hepatitis, Addison's disease, Sjögren's syndrome, rheumatoid arthritis and SLE have also been associated[3,62].

Recurrent infections can also be associated with IgA deficiency. They are clearly less severe than those seen in patients with 'common variable' immunodeficiency (CVID), but in both forms of antibody deficiency the patients usually start with upper respiratory tract infections[63]. However, the morphological changes in the nasal mucosa were much more severe in those with CVID, who also suffered from chronic rhinosinusitis[64]. Mucociliary function was less affected in the IgA deficient patients, presumably because of less infections. Lower respiratory tract infections started a few years after the onset of the upper tract infection, but were less common among the IgA deficient patients than in those with CVID. Patients with recurrent bronchopneumonia and IgA deficiency tended to neglect and understate their upper respiratory infections[63,65].

An increased risk of chronic lung function impairment was noted among both IgA deficient patients with low levels of IgG2 or IgG3[66] and among those with IgG subclass deficiency who also lacked IgA[67], indicating that the IgG subclass as well as the IgG deficiency may contribute to the risk.

A few patients with isolated IgA deficiency have severe problems with recurrent infections and it would seem important to define this group and find better ways of treating and preventing lung damage.

The reason that IgA deficiency is not always followed by an increased frequency of infections may be due to compensatory increased IgM production in mucosal membranes[68-70], which is transported into secretions. Mellander et al. showed that IgM antibodies to E. coli and poliovirus were significantly elevated above normal in the nasal secretions of IgA deficient individuals who were not prone to infections[71]. In contrast, the levels were not significantly elevated in those with IgA deficiency and frequent infections.

It is interesting that IgA deficient patients who have an increased production of IgD in their nasal mucosa had almost as many infections as those who had very few mucosal immunocytes of any isotype[70]. This is probably because IgD, in contrast to IgM, is not transferred across the epithelium. The available information suggests a close relationship between the number of immunocytes producing IgM and the severity of infections in the IgA deficient patients. This is reminiscent of CVID patients who predominantly have infections in the respiratory tract where they are notably deficient in mucosal immunocytes[72]. In contrast, they have fewer infections in the gastrointestinal tract, where there are usually many more mucosal lymphoid cells producing immunoglobulins[73]. Klemola and Savilathi[74] recently found significantly increased numbers of intraepithelial lymphocytes in the intestinal mucosa of IgA deficient individuals, but no difference in the relative numbers of T cells or T cell subpopulations compared to controls. A striking increase of goblet cells was noted in the nasal mucosa of IgA deficient patients as compared to normals, or to patients with CVID who often lacked such cells altogether[75]. It was suggested from these studies that the appearance of the goblet cells was T lymphocyte dependent, but it was not clear whether their increase was secondary to the frequent infections in these IgA deficient patients. The submucosal glands were not increased in IgA deficiency, but were in CVID. This is possibly a compensatory mechanism, which cannot be similarly T lymphocyte dependent, since the increase could be seen also in those CVID patients who showed evidence of impaired T lymphocyte function and had no goblet cells in their nasal mucosa.

The response to vaccination with meningococcal A and C carbohydrate capsules in infection-prone IgA deficient patients with normal IgG subclasses provides further evidence of immunological aberrations. Fewer patients than normal responded, and among the responders a few produced excessive amounts of antibodies[76]. It has recently been observed that peroral vaccination with live poliovirus vaccine in IgA deficient individuals led to prolonged faecal excretion of the virus compared to normal subjects[77].

These findings illustrate that individuals with IgA deficiency can be grouped into those with a compensated deficiency and no increase in the frequency of infections and those with repeated infections and a risk of chronic lung disease, especially in the presence of IgG subclass deficiency[66, 67]. There is also a subgroup with an increase in the mucosal IgD-producing cells. An increase in goblet cell numbers may help mucosal defence or may just be a consequence of frequent infections. Further analyses of these parameters may help us select those patients who need treatment before they develop lung damage.

CLINICAL SIGNIFICANCE OF IgG SUBCLASS DEFICIENCIES

Although IgG subclass deficiency was first described in 1968[6], the clinical significance is still unclear. Determination of serum IgG, IgA and IgM levels has long been routinely performed in patients with increased susceptibility to infections. Isolated subclass deficiencies may be present in spite of normal or even increased total IgG levels. With the availability of monoclonal reagents, standardized assays can be performed, although the determinations may still not be optimal[78].

Some patients with IgG subclass deficiency have frequent upper respiratory tract infections, otitis media, sinusitis, bronchopulmonary infections, osteomyelitis, meningitis, group B streptococcal septicaemia, urinary tract infections, episodes of fever and skin infections (recurrent herpes simplex, erysipelas). Moreover, muscle diseases, bronchial asthma, diabetes mellitus type I, Henoch Schönlein's purpura, chronic granulomatous disease, Bechterew and Friedreich's ataxia have been reported in association with IgG subclass deficiencies[9, 10, 79-81]. Low levels of the IgG subclasses can also be found among patients with various other immunodeficiencies, such as IgA deficiency and ataxia-telangiectasia[13, 18, 30]. Two patients with IgG2 deficiency and defective expression of MHC class II have been described[82].

Vaccination with polysaccharide antigens has demonstrated that IgG2 antibody responses vary according to the prevaccination level of IgG2[83]. This is also true for antibodies to the capsules of *Haemophilus influenzae* and pneumococci[84, 85], whether or not they are conjugated to a carrier protein[76, 86]. Patients with ataxia-telangiectasia and IgG2-IgG4 deficiency also respond poorly to pneumococcal vaccines[87].

Vasculitis occurs among subclass deficient individuals[82, 88], with the severity of the vasculitis varying from mild cutaneous lesions to polyvisceral involvement. The symptoms were exacerbated by infections and a dramatic improvement was observed following injection of immunoglobulin (Ig).

Diarrhoea was common in one study of IgG2 deficient patients, but this may be a symptom of infection since *Pseudomonas* was frequently found in the faeces, and there was a dramatic improvement after Ig prophylaxis[82]. However, we have observed a high frequency of IgG3 deficiency among patients with food intolerance and diarrhoea. The symptoms were not related to an abnormal faecal flora. Several authors have seen an association between autoimmune cytopenia and IgG subclass deficiency[82, 90].

There have been recent reports of a reduction in the seizures in children with intractable epilepsy following high-dose intravenous immunoglobulin therapy[91-93]. In the largest study, IgG2 deficiency was detected in six out of 12 children[93, 94]. All but one of the six deficient children responded to Ig therapy with a gradual decrease in the number of seizures and almost complete disappearance after 6 months. After reducing the dose of immunoglobulin, EEG abnormalities reappeared and then disappeared after the dose was increased. The mechanisms behind these remarkable observations are unknown.

Subnormal IgG subclass levels have also been reported among healthy individuals[95, 96], suggesting that subclass deficiency is either a cofactor for disease or is sometimes associated with another, as yet unidentified, defect. It can be seen that a broad variety of diseases and symptoms have been reported in association with IgG subclass deficiency. Further research is needed to improve our understanding of these associations, and how they relate to immunopathology. The most important issue for clinicians is to decide which patients need treatment with Ig replacement therapy; such decisions at the moment are largely based on intuition.

TREATMENT OF PATIENTS WITH DEFICIENCIES OF IgG SUBCLASSES AND OF IgA

The main principle is that acute infection should be actively treated and recurrent and chronic infections should be prevented. An important task is to prevent chronic inflammatory changes in the lungs[66, 67, 97].

Antibiotics should be liberally used during acute infections, and this should be impressed on all those regularly attending the patient. Long-term treatment may be occasionally required for chronic productive cough. In our experience trimethoprim, with or without sulphonamide, is very effective Regular postural lung drainage is important if there is evidence of chronic infection. Positive expiratory pressure during drainage is useful in those with bronchiectasis, as mucociliary function is often impaired[64, 98]. Some patients may have a minor reversible obstructive component, requiring β_2-stimulators. Mucociliary activity can also be increased by β_2-stimulators[99]. Mucolytic therapy may be valuable in patients with chronic bronchitis[99] using acetylcystein[100] and nebulized saline. The nasal mucosa is sometimes helped by regular washing with saline. The eyes, which are often neglected, may also benefit from regular saline washes.

Immunoglobulin prophylaxis for infections has not yet been tested in controlled studies of patients with IgG subclass deficiencies. However, 38 patients with low levels of one or more IgG subclasses received Ig prophylaxis with at least $25 \, \text{mg kg}^{-1} \, \text{week}^{-1}$ for more than 1500 patient-months; a retrospective analysis showed a significant decrease ($p<0.01$) in days on antibiotic treatment and episodes of infection[67]. Such a good effect had previously been noted in the family with IgG2 and IgG4 deficiency by Oxelius in 1974[10]. There is also an impression that immunoglobulin prophylaxis may be helpful in patients with combined IgA–IgG subclass deficiency[13, 66, 67].

Immunoglobulin prophylaxis was very helpful in patients with IgG deficiency and intractable epilepsy[93, 94]. In a preliminary study, diarrhoea in patients with food intolerance and associated IgG3 deficiency also improved on Ig therapy (Bengtsson *et al.*, personal communication). Some clinicians consider that Ig therapy is contraindicated in IgA deficiency because of the possibility of anaphylactic reactions due to anti-IgA antibodies. However, it is possible to give Ig prophylaxis to patients with combined low levels of Ig subclasses and IgA using an Ig with a very low content of IgA[101−103]. Even patients with anti-IgA antibodies and a history of reactions can be treated with such preparation.

One patient with IgA deficiency who had had six uneventful intravenous infusions had an anaphylactic reaction during the seventh. His titre of serum anti-IgA had increased steadily over the previous few months. It was suggested that this patient's anti-IgA was one of the IgE class[103], but we have not been able to confirm this on the same sample[102].

In patients with immunodeficiency and chronic or recurrent bacterial conjunctivitis, we and others (MacDowall, personal communication) have noted that local application in the eye of immunoglobulin preparations suitable for intramuscular use can be helpful.

ACKNOWLEDGEMENTS

Our studies referred to in this review were supported by grants from the Swedish Medical Research Council (No. 215), the Swedish Board for Technical Development and the Ellen, Walter and Lennart Hesselman Foundation.

References

1. Bruton, O. C. (1952). Agammaglobulinemia. *Pediatrics*, **9**, 722–8
2. Rockey, J. H., Hanson, L. Å., Heremans, J. F. and Kunkel, H. G. (1964). Beta-2A aglobulinemia in two healthy men. *J. Lab. Clin. Med.*, **63**, 205–12
3. Hanson, L. Å., Björkander, J. and Oxelius, V.-A. (1983). Selective IgA deficiency. In Chandra, R. K. (ed.) *Primary and Secondary Immunodeficiency Disorders.* pp. 62–84. (Edinburgh: Churchill Livingstone)
4. Buckley, R. H. and Dees, S. C. (1969). Correlation of milk precipitins with IgA deficiency. *N. Engl. J. Med.*, **281**, 465–9
5. Cunningham-Rundles, C., Pudifin, D. J., Armstrong, D. and Good, R. A. (1980). Selective IgA deficiency and neoplasia. *Vox Sang.*, **38**, 61–7
6. Terry, W. D. (1968). Variations in the subclasses of IgG. In Bergsma, D. (ed.) *Immunology Deficiency Diseases in Man.* Birth Defects: Original Article Series. Vol. 4, pp. 357–69. (New York: Liss)
7. Rivat, L., Ropartz, C., Burtin, P. and Karitzky, D. (1969). Abnormalities in synthesis of some subclasses of gammaG in a family with two cases of ataxia telangiectasia. *Vox Sang.*, **17**, 5–10
8. Leddy, J. P., Deitchman, J. and Bakemeier, R. F. (1970). IgG subclasses: measurement by radioimmunoassay in normal and hypogammaglobulinemic sera. *Arthr. Rheumat.*, **13**, 331–2
9. Schur, P. H., Borel, H., Gelfand, E. W., Alper, C. A. and Rosen, F. S. (1970). Selective gamma-G globulin deficiencies in patients with recurrent pyogenic infections. *N. Engl. J. Med.*, **283**, 631–4
10. Oxelius, V.-A. (1974). Chronic infections in a family with hereditary deficiency of IgG2 and IgG4. *Clin. Exp. Immunol.*, **17**, 19–27
11. Yount, W. J., Utsinger, P. D., Gatti, R. A. and Good, R. A. (1974). Immunoglobulin classes, IgG subclasses, Gm genetic markers, and clq following bone marrow transplantation in X-linked combined immunodeficiency. *J. Pediatr.*, **84**, 193–9
12. Hanson, L. Å., Söderström, T. and Oxelius, V.-A. (eds.) (1986). *Immunoglobulin Subclass Deficiencies.* Monogr. Allergy, Vol. 20. (Basel: Karger)
13. Oxelius, V.-A., Laurell, A.-B., Lindquist, B., Golebiowska, H., Axelsson, U., Björkander, J. and Hanson, L. Å. (1981). IgG subclasses in selective IgA deficiency. Common occurrence of IgG2-IgA deficiency. *N. Engl. J. Med.*, **304**, 1476–7
14. Ugazio, A. G., Out, T. A., Plebani, A., Duse, M., Monafo, V., Nespoli, L. and Burgio, G. R. (1983). Recurrent infections in children with selective IgA deficiency: association with IgG2 and IgG4 deficiency. In Wedgwood, R. J., Rosen, F. S. and Paul, N. W. (eds.) *Primary Immunodeficiency Diseases.* Birth Defects: Original Article Series, Vol. 19, pp. 169–71. (New York: Liss)
15. Cunningham-Rundles, C., Oxelius, V.-A. and Good, R. A. (1983). IgG2 and IgG3 subclass deficiencies in selective IgA deficiency in the United States. In Wedgwood, R. J., Rosen, F. S. and Paul, N. W. (eds.) *Primary Immunodeficiency Diseases.* Birth Defects: Original Article Series, Vol. 19, pp. 173–5. (New York: Liss)
16. Plebani, A., Monafo, V., Avanzini, M. A., Ugazio, A. G. and Burgio, G. R. (1986). Relationship between IgA and IgG subclass deficiencies: a reappraisal. In Hanson, L. Å., Söderström, T. and Oxelius, V.-A. (eds.) *Immunoglobulin Subclass Deficiencies.* Monogr. Allergy, Vol. 20, pp. 171–8. (Basel: Karger)
17. Rivat-Peran, L., Buriot, D., Sailer, J.-P., Rivat, C., Dumitresco, S.-M. and Griscelli, C. (1981). Immunoglobulins in ataxia-telangiectasia: evidence for IgG4 and IgG2 subclass deficiencies. *Clin. Immunol. Immunopathol.*, **20**, 99–110

18. Oxelius, V.-A., Berkel, A. I. and Hanson, L. Å. (1982). IgG2 deficiency in ataxia-telangiectasia. *N. Engl. J. Med.*, **306**, 515-17
19. Hammarström, L., Grubb, R., Oxelius, V.-A., Persson, U., Smith, C. I. E. and Svejgaard, A. (1986). Concomitant deficiency of IgG4 and IgE in IgA-deficient donors with high titres of anti-IgA. In Hanson, L. Å., Söderström, T. and Oxelius, V.-A. (eds.) *Immunoglobulin Subclass Deficiencies.* Monogr. Allergy, Vol. 20, pp. 234-5. (Bassel: Karger)
20. Bajtai, G., Ambrus, M., Paál, M., Nagy, J. and Deák, Gy. (1975). Hepatitis-B antigenaemia associated with progressive cirrhosis and membranous glomerulonephritis. *Lancet*, **1**, 102-3
21. Ambrus, M., Hernádi, E. and Bajtai, G. (1977). Prevalence of HLA-A1 and HLA-B8 antigens in selective IgA deficiency. *Clin. Immunol. Immunopathol.*, **7**, 311-14
22. Smith, W. I., Rabin, B. S., Huellmantel, A., van Thiel, D. H. and Drash, A. (1978). Immunopathology of juvenile-onset diabetes mellitus. I. IgA deficiency and juvenile diabetes. *Diabetes*, **27**, 1092-7
23. Hammarström, L., Axelsson, U., Björkander, J., Hanson, L. Å., Möller, E, and Smith, C. I. E. (1984). HLA antigens in selective IgA deficiency: distribution in healthy donors and patients with recurrent respiratory tract infections. *Tissue Antigens*, **24**, 35-9
24. Feingold, M. and Schwartz, R. S. (1968). IgA and partial deletions of chromosome 18. *Lancet*, **2**, 1086
25. Claman, H. N., Merrill, D. A., Peakman, D. and Robinson, A. (1970). Isolated severe gamma A deficiency: immunoglobulin levels, clinical disorders, and chromosome studies. *J. Lab. Clin. Med.*, **75**, 307-15
26. Ogata, K., Iinuma, K., Kamimura, K., Morinaga, R. and Kato, J. (1977). A case report of a presumptive +i(18p) associated with serum IgA deficiency. *Clin. Genet.*, **11**, 184-8
27. Muñoz-López, F., Martinez, F. B. and Mateos, M. A. M. (1977). Selective IgA deficiency. Immunologic and cytogenetic studies. *Allergol. Immunopathol.*, **V**, 671-6
28. Smith, C. I. E. and Hammarström, L. (1986). Detection of immunoglobulin genes in individuals with immunoglobulin class or subclass deficiency. Evidence for a pretranslational defect. In Hanson, L. Å., Söderström, T. and Oxelius, V.-A. (eds.) *Immunoglobulin Subclass Deficiencies.* Monogr. Allergy. Vol. 20, pp. 18-25. (Basel: Karger)
29. Smith, C. I. E. and Hammarström, L. (1986). Transcription of immunoglobulin C-alfa-genes in individuals with IgA deficiency. In Vossen, J. and Griscelli, C. (eds.) *Progress in Immunodeficiency Research and Therapy.* Vol. II, pp. 255-60. (Amsterdam: Excerpta Medica)
30. Oxelius, V.-A., Hanson, L. Å., Björkander, J., Hammarström, L. and Sjöholm, A. (1986). IgG3 deficiency: common in obstructive lung disease. Hereditary in families with immunodeficiency and autoimmune disease. In Hanson, L. Å., Söderström, T. and Oxelius, V.-A. (eds.) *Immunoglobulin Subclass Deficiencies.* Monogr. Allergy, Vol. 20, pp. 106-15. (Basel: Karger)
31. Yount, W. J., Kunkel, H. G. and Litwin, S. D. (1967). Studies of the Vi (gamma 2c) subgroup of gammaglobulin. A relationship between concentration and genetic type among normal individuals. *J. Exp. Med.*, **125**, 177-90
32. Oxelius, V.-A. (1979). IgG subclass levels in infancy and childhood. *Acta Paediatr. Scand.*, **68**, 23-7
33. Grubb, R., Hallberg, T., Hammarström, L., Oxelius, V.-A., Smith, C. I. E., Söderström, R. and Söderström, T. (1986). Correlation between deficiency of immunoglobulin subclass G3 and Gm allotype. *Acta Pathol. Microbiol. Immunol. Scand. Sect. C.*, **94**, 187-91
34. Lefranc, M.-P., Lefranc, G., DeLange, G., Out, T. A., van den Broek, P. J., van Nieuwoop, J., Radl, J., Helal, A. N., Chaabani, H., van Loghem, E. and Rabbitts, T. H. (1983). Instability of the human immunoglobulin heavy chain constant region locus indicated by different inherited chromosomal deletions. *Mol. Biol. Med.*, **1**, 207-17
35. Migone, N., Oliviero, S., deLange, G., Delacroix, D. L., Boschis, D., Altruda, F., Silengo, L., De Marchi, M. and Carbonara, A. O. (1984). Multiple gene deletions within the human immunoglobulin heavy-chain cluster. *Proc. Natl. Acad. Sci. USA.*, **81**, 5811-15
36. Savilathi, E. and Pelkonen, P. (1979). Clinical findings and intestinal immunoglobulins in children with partial IgA deficiency. *Acta Paediatr. Scand.*, **68**, 513-19
37. Østergaard, P. A. (1980). Clinical and immunological features of transient IgA deficiency in children. *Clin. Exp. Immunol.*, **40**, 561-5

38. Buckley, R. H. (1975). Clinical and immunologic features of selective IgA deficiency. In Bergsma, D. (ed.) *Immunodeficiency in Man and in Animals*. Birth Defects: Original Articles Series, Vol. II, pp. 134-42. (New York: Liss)

39. Plebani, A., Ugazio, A. G., Monafo, V. and Burgio G. R. (1986). Clinical heterogeneity and reversibility of selective immunoglobulin A deficiency in 80 children. *Lancet*, 1, 829-31

40. Gillon, J., Barclay, G. R., Yap, P. L. and Ferguson, A. (1986). Food antibodies, intestinal permeability and HLA status in IgA deficient blood donors identified by a new rapid screening test. *Clin. Allergy*, 16, 583-8

41. Söderström, T., Söderström, R., Bengtsson, U., Björkander, J., Hellstrand, K., Holm, J. and Hanson, L. Å. (1986). Clinical and immunological evaluation of patients low in single or multiple IgG subclasses. In Hanson, L. Å., Söderström, T. and Oxelius, V.-A. (eds.) *Immunoglobulin Subclass Deficiencies*. Monogr. Allergy, Vol. 20, pp. 135-42. (Basel: Karger)

42. Söderström, T., Söderström, R., Avanzini, A., Brandtzaeg, P., Karlsson, G. and Hanson, L. Å. (1987). Immunoglobulin G subclass deficiencies. *Int. Archs. Allergy Appl. Immunol.*, 82, 476-80

43. Smith, T. F. and Bain, R. P. (1986). IgG subclasses in children with chronic chest symptoms. In Hanson, L. Å., Söderström, T. and Oxelius, V.-A. (eds.) *Immunoglobulin Subclass Deficiencies*. Monogr. Allergy, Vol. 20, pp. 119-27. (Basel: Karger)

44. Anderson, U., Bird, A. G., Britton, S. and Palacios, R. (1981). Humoral and cellular immunity in humans studied at the cell level from birth to two years of age. *Immunol. Rev.*, 57, 5-38

45. Hammarström, L., Lefranc, G., Lefranc, M. P., Persson, M. A. A. and Smith, C. I. E. (1986). Aberrant pattern of anti-carbohydrate antibodies in immunoglobulin class of subclass-deficient donors. In Hanson, L. Å., Söderström, T. and Oxelius, V.-A. (eds.) *Immunoglobulin Subclass Deficiencies*. Monogr. Allergy, Vol. 20, pp. 50-6. (Basel: Karger)

46. Söderström, T., Söderström, R. and Hanson, L. Å. (1988). Low immunoglobulin G subclass levels as an indicator of immune dysfunction. Medica Hoechst, Vol. 21 (Stuttgart: Schattauer Verlag) (In press)

47. Quinti, I., Papetti, C., Testi, R., Bonomo, R. and Aiuti, F. (1986). IgG subclass deficiency in adults: a clinical and immunological study. In Hanson, L. Å., Söderström, T. and Oxelius, V.-A. (eds.) *Immunoglobulin Subclass Deficiencies*. Monogr. Allergy, Vol. 20, pp. 143-48. (Basel: Karger)

48. Hanson, L. Å. and Brandtzaeg, P. (1988). The mucosal defense system. In Stiehm, R. T. (ed.) *Immunological Diseases in Infants and Children*. 3rd edn. (Philadelphia: Saunders) (In press)

49. Griffiss, J. M. and Bertram, M. A. (1977). Immunoepidemiology of meningococcal disease in military recruits. II. Blocking of serum bactericidal activity by circulating IgA early in the course of invasive disease. *J. Infect. Dis.*, 136, 733-9

50. Yount, W. J., Dorner, M. M., Kunkel, H. G. and Kabat, E. A. (1968). Studies on human antibodies. VI. Selective variations in subgroup composition and genetic markers. *J. Exp. Med.*, 127, 633-46

51. Söderström, T., Enskog, A., Samuelsson, B. E. and Cedergren, B. (1984). Immunoglobulin subclass (IgG3) restriction of anti-p and anti-p^k antibodies in patients of the rare p blood group. *J. Immunol.*, 134, 1-3

52. Sundquist, V.-A., Linde, A. and Wahren, B. (1984). Virus-specific immunoglobulin G subclasses in herpes simplex and varicella-zoster virus infections. *J. Clin. Microbiol.*, 20, 94-8

53. Gilljam, G., Sundquist, V.-A. Linde, A., Philstedt, P., Eklund, A. E. and Wahren, B. (1985). Sensitive analytic ELISAs for subclass virus IgG. *J. Virol. Meth.*, 10, 203-14

54. Linde, A. (1985). Subclass distribution of rubella virus-specific immunoglobulin G. *J. Clin. Microbiol.*, 21, 117-21

55. Husby, S., Oxelius, V.-A., Teisner, B., Jensenius, J. C. and Svehag, S.-E. (1985). Humoral immunity to dietary antigens in healthy adults: occurrence, isotype and IgG subclass distribution of serum antibodies to protein antigens. *Int. Arch. Allergy Appl. Immunol.*, 77, 416-22

56. Shakib, F. and Stanworth, D. R. (1980). Human IgG subclasses in health and disease. I. *La Ricerca Clin. Lab.*, **10**, 463-79
57. Shakib, F. and Stanworth, D. R. (1980). Human IgG subclasses in health and disease. II. *La Ricerca Clin. Lab.*, **10**, 561-80
58. Björksten, B. (1983). Doest breast-feeding prevent the development of allergy? *Immunol. Today*, **4**, 215-17
59. van der Giessen, M., Reerink-Brongers, E. E. and Algra-van Veen, T. (1976). Quantitation of Ig classes and IgG subclasses in sera of patients with a variety of immunoglobulin deficiencies and their relatives. *Clin. Immunol. Immunopathol.*, **5**, 388-98
60. Iskander, R., Das, P. K. and Aalberse, R. C. (1981). IgG4 antibodies in Egyptian patients with schistosomiasis. *Int. Arch. Allergy Appl. Immunol.*, **66**, 200-7
61. Djurup, R. (1985). The subclass nature and clinical significance of the IgG antibody response in patients undergoing allergen-specific immunotherapy. *Allergy*, **40**, 469-86
62. Ammann, A. J. and Hong, R. (1980). Disorders of the IgA system. In Stiehm, R. T. and Fulginiti, V. (eds.) *Immunologic Disorders in Infants and Children*. 2nd edn., pp. 260-73. (Philadelphia: Saunders)
63. Karlsson G., Petruson, B., Björkander, J. and Hanson, L. Å. (1985). Infections of the nose and paranasal sinuses in adult patients with immunodeficiency. *Arch. Otolaryngol.*, **111**, 290-3
64. Karlsson, G., Hansson, H.-A., Petruson, B. and Björkander, J. (1985). The nasal mucosa in immunodeficiency. *Acta Otolaryngol.*, **100**, 456-69
65. Karlsson, G. (1986). *The Nasal Mucosa in Humoral Immunodeficiency*. Thesis. (Göteborg: University of Göteborg)
66. Björkander, J., Bake, B., Oxelius, V.-A. and Hanson, L. Å. (1985). Impaired lung function in patients with IgA deficiency and low levels of IgG2 or IgG3. *N. Engl. J. Med.*, **313**, 720-4
67. Björkander, J., Bengtsson, U., Oxelius, V.-A. and Hanson, L. Å. (1986). Symptoms in patients with lowered levels of IgG subclasses, with or without IgA deficiency, and effects of immunoglobulin prophylaxis. In Hanson, L. Å., Söderström, T. and Oxelius, V.-A. (eds.) *Immunoglobulin Subclass Deficiencies*. Monogr. Allergy, Vol. 20, pp. 157-63. (Basel: Karger)
68. Brandtzaeg, P., Fjellanger, I. and Gjeruldsen, S. T. (1968). Immunoglobulin M: local synthesis and selective secretion in patients with immunoglobulin A deficiency. *Science*, **160**, 789-91
69. Brandtzaeg, P., Kett, K., Rognum, T. O., Söderström, R., Björkander, J., Söderström, T., Petrusson, B. and Hanson, L. Å. (1986). Distribution of mucosal IgA and IgG subclass-producing immunocytes and alterations in various disorders. In Hanson, L. Å., Söderström, T. and Oxelius, V.-A. (eds.) *Immunoglobulin Subclass Deficiencies*. Monogr. Allergy, Vol. 20, pp. 179-94. (Basel: Karger)
70. Brandtzaeg, P., Karlsson, G., Hansson, G., Petruson, B., Björkander, J. and Hanson, L. Å. (1988). The clinical condition of IgA-deficient patients is related to the proportion of IgD- and IgM-producing cells in their nasal mucosa. *Clin. Exp. Immunol.*, **67**, 626-36
71. Mellander, L., Björkander, J., Carlsson, B. and Hanson, L. Å. (1986). Secretory antibodies in IgA-deficient and immunosuppressed individuals. *J. Clin. Immunol.*, **6**, 284-91
72. Karlsson, G., Brandtzaeg, P., Hansson, G., Petruson, B., Björkander, J. and Hanson, L. Å. (1988). Humoral immunity in nasal mucosa of patients with common variable immunodeficiency. *J. Clin. Immunol.*, **7**, 29-36
73. Broom, B. C., de la Concha, E. G., Webster, A. D. B., Loewi, G. and Asherson, G. L. (1975). Dichotomy between immunoglobulin synthesis by cells in gut and blood of patients with hypogammaglobulinaemia. *Lancet*, **2**, 253-6
74. Klemola, T. and Savilathi, E. (1986). T cells and T cell subpopulations in the jejunum of IgA deficient persons. In Vossen, J. and Griscelli, C. (eds.) *Progress in Immunodeficiency Research and Therapy*. Vol. II, pp. 269-77. (Amsterdam: Excerpta Medica)
75. Karlsson, G., Hansson, H.-A., Petruson, B., Björkander, J. and Hanson, L. Å. (1985). Goblet cell number in the nasal mucosa relates to cell-mediated immunity in patients with antibody deficiency syndromes. *Int. Arch. Allergy Appl. Immunol.*, **78**, 86-91
76. Avanzini, M. A., Söderström, T., Schneerson, R., Robbins, J. B., Söderström, R.,

Björkander, J. and Hanson, L. Å. (1986). The heterogeneity of the antibody response in patients with IgG subclass deficiency is reflected on vaccination. In Vossen, J. and Griscelli, C. (eds.) *Progress in Immunodeficiency Research and Therapy*. Vol. II, pp. 241-5. (Amsterdam: Excerpta Medica)

77. Savilathi, E., Klemola, T., Hovi, T., Carlson, B., Stenvik, M., Mellander, L. and Tiainen P. (1986). IgA deficient persons excrete attenuated vaccine viruses longer than controls. In Vossen, J. and Griscelli, C. (eds.) *Progress in Immunodeficiency Research and Therapy*. Vol. II, pp. 261-7. (Amsterdam: Excerpta Medica)

78. Jefferis, R. (1986). Human IgG subclass-specific epitopes recognised by murine monoclonal antibodies. In Hanson, L. Å., Söderström, T. and Oxelius, V.-A. (eds.) *Immunoglobulin Subclass Deficiencies*. Monogr. Allergy, Vol. 20, pp. 26-33. (Basel: Karger)

79. Bass, J. L., Nuss, R., Mehta, K. A., Morganelli, P. and Bennet, L. (1983). Recurrent meningococcemia associated with IgG2-subclass deficiency. *N. Engl. J. Med.*, **309**, 430

80. Oxelius, V.-A. (1979). Quantitative and qualitative investigations of serum IgG subclasses in immunodeficiency diseases. *Clin. Exp. Immunol.*, **36**, 112-16

81. Oxelius, V.-A. (1984). Immunoglobulin G (IgG) subclasses and human disease. *Am. J. Med.*, **76** (3A), 7-18

82. Bremard-Oury, C., Aucouturier, P., Debré, M., Preud'homme, J. L. and Griscelli, C. (1986). Immunoglobulin G subclasses in patients with immunodeficiencies. In Hanson, L. Å., Söderström, T. and Oxelius, V.-A. (eds.) *Immunoglobulin Subclass Deficiencies*. Monogr. Allergy, Vol. 20, pp. 75-9. (Basel: Karger)

83. Siber, G. R., Schur, P. H., Aisenberg, A. C., Weitzman, S. A. and Schiffman, G. (1980). Correlation between serum IgG-2 concentrations and the antibody response to bacterial polysaccharide antigens. *N. Engl. J. Med.*, **303**, 178-82

84. Umetsu, D. T., Ambrosino, D. M., Quinti, I., Siber, G. R. and Geha, R. S. (1985). Recurrent sinopulmonary infection and impaired antibody response to bacterial capsular polysaccharide antigen in children with selective IgG subclass deficiency. *N. Engl. J. Med.*, **313**, 1247-51

85. Umetsu, D. T., Ambrosino, D. M. and Geha, R. S. (1986). Children with selective IgG subclass deficiency and recurrent sinopulmonary infection: impaired response to bacterial capsular polysaccharide antigens. In Hanson, L. Å., Söderström, T. and Oxelius, V.-A. (eds.) *Immunoglobulin Subclass Deficiencies*. Monogr. Allergy, Vol. 20, pp. 57-61. (Basel: Karger)

86. Söderström, T., Avanzini, A., Björkander, J., Söderström, R., Robbins, J. B. and Hanson, L. Å. (1988). Antibody response against *Haemophilus influenzae* type b and tetanus toxoid in patients with IgG subclass deficiency. (In manuscript)

87. Berkel, A. I. (1986). Studies of IgG subclasses in ataxia-telangiectasia patients. In Hanson, L. Å., Söderström, T. and Oxelius, V.-A. (eds.) *Immunoglobulin Subclass Deficiencies*. Monogr. Allergy, Vol. 20, pp. 100-5. (Basel: Karger)

88. Bremard-Oury, C., Aucouturier, P., Le Deist, F., Debré, M., Preud'homme, J. L. and Griscelli, C. (1986). The spectrum of IgG2 deficiencies. In Vossen, J. and Griscelli, C. (eds.) *Progress in Immunodeficiency Research and Therapy*. Vol. II, pp. 235-9. (Amsterdam: Excerpta Medica)

89. Söderström, T., Söderström, R., Bengtsson, U., Björkander, J., Hellstrand, K., Holm, J. and Hanson, L. Å. (1986). Clinical and immunological evaluation of patients low in single or multiple IgG subclasses. In Hanson, L. Å., Söderström, T. and Oxelius, V.-A. (eds.) *Immunoglobulin Subclass Deficiencies*. Monogr. Allergy, Vol. 20, pp. 135-42. (Basel: Karger)

90. Bussel, J., Morell, A. and Skvaril, F. (1986). IgG2 deficiency in autoimmune cytopenias. In Hanson, L. Å., Söderström, T. and Oxelius, V.-A. (eds.) *Immunoglobulin Subclass Deficiencies*. Monogr. Allergy, Vol. 20, pp. 116-18. (Basel: Karger)

91. Ariizumi, M., Shiihara, H., Hibio, S., Ryo, S., Baba, K., Ogawa, K., Suzuki, Y. and Momoki, T. (1983). High dose gammaglobulin for intractable childhood epilepsy. *Lancet*, **2**, 162-3

92. Sandstedt, P., Kostulas, V. and Larsson, L. E. (1984). Intravenous gammaglobulin for post-encephalitic epilepsy. *Lancet*, **2**, 1154-5

93. Duse, M., Tiberti, S., Plebani, A., Avanzini, M. A., Gardenghi, M., Menegati, E.,

Monafo, V. and Ugazio, A. G. (1986). IgG2 deficiency and intractable epilepsy of childhood. In Hanson, L. Å., Söderström, T. and Oxelius, V.-A. (eds.) *Immunoglobulin Subclass Deficiencies.* Monogr. Allergy, Vol. 20, pp. 128-34. (Basel: Karger)

94. Duse, M., Tiberti, S., Menegati, E., Plebani, A., Vertua, G., Gardenghi, M. and Ugazio, A. G. (1986). Intractable childhood epilepsy and IgG2 deficiency: evidence for a dose dependent therapeutic effect of intravenous gammaglobulin. In Vossen, J. and Griscelli, C. (eds.) *Progress in Immunodeficiency Research and Therapy.* Vol. II, pp. 205-10. (Amsterdam: Excerpta Medica)

95. Lefranc, M.-P., Lefranc, G. and Rabbits, T. H. (1982). Inherited deletion of immunoglobulin heavy chain constant region genes in normal human individuals. *Nature (London)*, **300**, 760-2

96. Hammarström, L. and Smith, C. I. E. (1983). IgG2 deficiency in a healthy blood donor: concomitant lack of IgG2, IgA and IgE immunoglobulins and specific anti-carbohydrate antibodies. *Clin. Exp. Immunol.*, **51**, 600-4

97. Björkander, J. (1985). *Antibody Deficiency Syndromes.* Thesis. (Göteborg: University of Göteborg)

98. Mossberg, B., Björkander, J., Afzelius, B. A. and Camner, P. (1982). Mucociliary clearance in patients with immunoglobulin deficiency. *Eur. J. Respir. Dis.*, **63**, 570-8

99. Mossberg, B., Strandberg, K., Philipson, K. and Camner, P. (1976). Tracheobronchial clearance and beta-adrenoreceptor stimulation in patients with chronic bronchitis. *Scand. J. Respir. Dis.*, **57**, 281-9

100. Boman, G., Bäcker, U., Larsson, S., Melander, B. and Wåhlander, L. (1983). Oral acetylcystein reduces exacerbation rate in chronic bronchitis: report of a trial organized by The Swedish Society for Pulmonary Diseases. *Eur. J. Respir: Dis.*, **64**, 405-15

101. Hanson, L. Å., Björkander, J., Ljunggren, C., Oxelius, V.-A. and Wadsworth, C. (1980). Problems with use of immunoglobulins in treatment of immunodeficient patients. In Alving, B. M. and Finlayson, J. S. (eds.) *Immunoglobulins: Characteristics and Uses of Intravenous Preparations.* pp. 151-9. (Washington: US Department of Health, and Human Services, DHHS Publication No. (FDA)-80-9005)

102. Björkander, J., Hammarström, L., Smith, C. I. E., Buckely, R. H., Cunningham-Rundles, C. and Hanson, L. Å. (1988). Immunoglobulin prophylaxis in patients with antibody deficiency syndromes and anti IgA. *J. Clin. Immunol.*, **7**, 8-15

103. Burks, A. W., Sampson, H. A. and Buckley, R. H. (1986). Anaphylactic reactions after gammaglobulin administration in patients with hypogammaglobulinemia. *N. Engl. J. Med.*, **314**, 560-4

6
Metabolic Causes of Immune Deficiency: Mechanisms and Treatment

B. J. M. ZEGERS AND J. W. STOOP

INTRODUCTION

In 1972, Dr Eloise R. Giblett, a haematologist, and her pediatrician colleagues described two unrelated children whose blood erythrocytes (and lymphocytes) lacked the purine enzyme adenosine deaminase (ADA)[1]. Both children suffered from a severe combined immune deficiency disease (SCID). At the same time a Danish group described two similar children with ADA deficiency associated with SCID[2]. It was suggested in these early reports that the defect in the immune system was caused by the enzyme deficiency. It was soon appreciated that the defect was inherited as an autosomal recessive, although it was some time before the enzyme deficiency could be mechanistically related to the immune deficiency. There was another major advance when Dr Giblett discovered another purine enzyme deficiency (purine nucleoside phosphorylase, PNP) in a patient with a selective cellular immune deficiency resembling the Nezelof syndrome[3]. The discovery of more PNP deficient patients showed that this was also an autosomal recessive disease[4,5]. Nowadays ADA and PNP deficiency are recognized as the primary cause of the associated immune deficiency.

There is one other well-defined molecular defect, i.e. deficiency of transcobalamine II (TC II), a transport protein for vitamin B12, which is associated with agammaglobulinaemia as well as with defects in the cells of the erythropoietic and myelopoietic lineage[6,7]. In addition, there are a number of metabolic or biochemical abnormalities which seem to be associated with immune deficiency. In these cases causal relationships are not yet definitely established (Table 6.1). Examples are hereditary orotic aciduria type I and biotin-dependent carboxylase deficiency[8,9]. The former may be associated with defects in cell-mediated immunity and the latter with clinical and immunological signs of a mild combined immunodeficiency disease (CID). Furthermore, acrodermatitis enteropathica, which is characterized by malabsorption, diarrhoea, eczema and recurrent respiratory tract infections,

Table 6.1 Metabolic defects associated with immune deficiency

	Immunodeficiency	*Association*
ADA deficiency	SCID	causal
PNP deficiency	cellular immunodeficiency	causal
TCII deficiency	agammaglobulinaemia	causal
Orotic aciduria type 1	cellular immunodeficiency in some cases	?
Biotin dependent carboxylase deficiency	CID in some cases	?
Zinc transport defect in acrodermatitis enteropathica	CID (variable)	?
Ecto-5' nucleotidase deficiency in Omenn's syndrome	CID	?

may be associated with CID and patients do respond to zinc therapy[10]. The association of a deficiency of the lymphocyte surface enzyme, ecto-5'-nucleotidase in patients with Omenn's syndrome (also called reticuloendotheliosis), which is consistently associated with CID, is still unexplained[11]. More recent findings suggest that there are defects in membrane signalling pathways of lymphocytes in some patients who clinically have combined immunodeficiency. Most of them have normal numbers of lymphocytes which fail to proliferate when activated with antigens or mitogens like phytohaemagglutinin. These lymphocyte defects may involve any one of the following events: ligand/receptor interactions; hydrolysis of phosphatidylinositol-bisphosphate by phospholipase-C which produces the second messenger diacylglycerol; Ca^{2+} mobilization from intracellular stores; and activation of protein kinase-C. However, such defects have not yet been properly documented.

CLINICAL AND IMMUNOLOGICAL CHARACTERISTICS OF ADA AND PNP DEFICIENCY

ADA-deficiency

Approximately 30–50% of patients with the autosomal recessive form of SCID have ADA–deficiency. Most ADA-patients develop the clinical symptoms of classical SCID in the first 6 months of life. A small number may remain asymptomatic until the second or third year of life because some residual immune function is retained. Clinically, these infants and young children fail to thrive and may suffer from diarrhoea and severe recurrent infections with bacteria, fungi, viruses and protozoa, particularly opportunistic pathogens like *Pneumocystis carinii*. The tonsillar tissue is not developed and their lymph nodes are atrophic. The thymus shadow is absent on the chest X-ray. Most ADA⁻ patients show characteristic skeletal abnormalities wich are due to abnormal growth of developing cartilage; and this may rarely cause short-limbed dwarfism. Neurological abnormalities, such as nystagmus and intermittent tremors of extremities and trunk, have been observed in a few ADA⁻ SCID patients; a causal relationship with the enzyme deficiency is questionable[5, 7].

ADA⁻SCID patients have profound lymphopenia with a marked decrease in T cell numbers and a mild or marked decrease in B cell counts. *In vitro* T cell proliferation following activation with mitogens and antigens is absent or severely decreased. Cutaneous delayed type hypersensitivity reactions are negative and skin grafts of unrelated donors are not rejected. Most patients are agammaglobulinaemic and do not produce specific antibodies. However, some patients, i.e. those with B lymphocytes, have low or even normal serum immunoglobulin levels and do make specific antibodies following infection or vaccination. A few patients develop fatal lymphoma of the B cell lineage[5, 7].

Despite thorough investigations, the variability in clinical and immuno-logical findings cannot be clearly related to the severity of the biochemical defect. An interesting characteristic of ADA deficiency is that the immunological defect becomes more severe with increasing age. This immunological involution was initially explained on the basis of the histological picture in the thymus glands of ADA⁻ SCID patients. These showed some differentiated epithelium, Hassall's corpuscles and large blood vessels, suggesting that they had previously been normal. Longitudinal studies in a few patients have shown a gradual fall in the circulating lymphocyte count with a deterioration of *in vivo* and *in vitro* T and B cell function with increasing age[5].

PNP deficiency

Patients with PNP deficiency show the clinical symptoms of a cellular immune deficiency. However, the susceptibility to infections is very variable; for instance some patients develop infections within the first year of life while others remain symptom free until 3 or more years. Some patients are prone to severe and recurrent respiratory infections but the severity of viral infections is the most striking. Lethal infections with *Varicella zoster*, measles and cytomegalovirus have been described, as well as generalized vaccinial infection following vaccination[4, 5, 7]. However, neither polio virus (type III) infection nor hepatitis B virus infection in one particular patient led to serious disease. Perhaps the lack of specific cellular immunity prevented a chronic hepatitis. Fatal lymphosarcoma, one of the B cell lineage and the other not delineated, has developed in two patients and graft versus host disease following transfusion with unirradiated blood was fatal in other patients[4, 5, 7].

Some patients have a megaloblastic bone marrow which may be associated with a macrocytic anaemia. Unlike the ADA deficiency, PNP deficient patients do not have skeletal abnormalities. However, neurologic abnormalities are common consisting of spastic tetra- or diparesis of extremities and spastic paresis of the trunk[4, 12]. These neurological features may even precede the onset of infections[13]. Neurological abnormalities, other than caused by infections, are uncommon in all types of SCID and CID. It is therefore likely that the central nervous system dysfunction is in some way related to the PNP deficiency. It has been argued that patients with PNP deficiency have an additional functional deficiency of hypoxanthine-guanine phosphoribosyl transferase (HGPRT), the enzyme which is deficient in the Lesch–Nyhan syndrome in which there is severe central nervous system dysfunction[14].

Characteristically, PNP deficient patients have severely impaired T lymphocyte function, as reflected by absent delayed type hypersensitivity, absent skin graft rejection and severely decreased or absent *in vitro* lymphocyte proliferation with mitogens and antigens[4,5,7].

A severe persistent lymphopenia of less than 400 lymphocytes/mm^3 is common, with low numbers of circulating T cells which usually express the T cell differentiation antigens CD3, CD4 and CD8. There are B lymphocytes in the peripheral blood, although they are usually low in number. Serum immunoglobulin levels are normal or increased and serum electrophoresis may show minor paraproteins superimposed on a polyclonal increase in gammaglobulins. Patients do synthesize specific antibodies following infection or vaccination, and sometimes these responses are exaggerated, suggesting a defect in the regulating of B cell function. However some patients with virus infections, such as *Varicella zoster*, only produce low titres of specific antibody which soon disappear[4,5,7]. No thymus shadow is visible on an X-ray of the thorax, and usually there is only little tonsillar tissue. Biopsies of lymph nodes show the characteristic picture of a selective T cell deficiency, i.e. intact germinal centres, the presence of plasma cells containing all major Ig isotypes but severe depletion of small T cells from the cortical areas. Pre-B cells, B cells and plasma cells are present in the bone marrow.

Autoimmune phenomena have occurred in some patients, such as the presence of antinuclear (ANA) antibodies associated with an SLE-like syndrome, autoimmune haemolytic anaemia associated with cytomegalovirus infection, and antibodies against kidney basement membrane associated with renal insufficiency in a Dutch patient. Rheumatoid factors and antinuclear antibodies, without evidence of autoimmune disease, have been found in the sera of a few patients. These autoimmune phenomena may be triggered by viral infections and some would argue that they are due to deficient T suppressor cell function[5].

Like ADA deficiency, PNP deficiency causes a progressive immuno-deficiency disease. At birth, circulating T lymphocyte numbers and *in vitro* T cell function may be normal, and then deteriorate during the first 6 months of life[4]. The thymus is usually hypoplastic, sometimes lacking Hassall's corpuscles, with some evidence of epithelial maturation.

Prevalence

More than 50 families have so far been described with ADA deficiency and concurrent SCID. There are a few healthy individuals, some of them members of the African Kung tribe who lack ADA in their erythrocytes but have sufficient ADA activity in lymphoid and fibroblast cells. However, one Caucasian infant with partial ADA deficiency showed impaired cellular immunity, suggesting that additional factors may determine the effect in the immune system[15,16]. About 22 patients from 15 families have been described with PNP deficiency. There are no descriptions of partial PNP deficiency without immune deficiency.

BIOCHEMICAL ABNORMALITIES

Adenosine deaminase (ADA; adenosine aminohydrolase, EC 3.5.4.4)

The purine enzyme, ADA, catalyses the deamination of adenosine and deoxyadenosine to inosine and deoxyinosine respectively (Figure 6.1). ADA activity is demonstrable in most body tissues. In blood, ADA is present in erythrocytes and leukocytes; among the lymphocytes T cells have higher activity than B cells. A comparison of T cells of different stages of maturation (i.e. thymocytes and peripheral blood T cells) showed that ADA activity is highest in immature thymocytes. In erythrocytes, the enzyme is present as a monomer of 38 kDa. In other cells and tissues the monomer is associated with the ADA-binding protein in a ratio of 2:1 respectively. Starch gel electrophoresis of red cell lysates shows polymorphism of ADA: three phenotypes can be detected[5,7], i.e. ADA1, ADA2 and the heterozygote ADA2-1. The human ADA locus is located[17] on chromosome 20.

It was thought initially that ADA$^-$ SCID patients had inactive or 'silent' alleles. However, messenger RNA can be detected and immunologically cross-reactive protein with little or no ADA activity is produced; often the protein is unstable and rapidly degraded[16]. Heterozygote parents have about 50% of ADA activity in their cells.

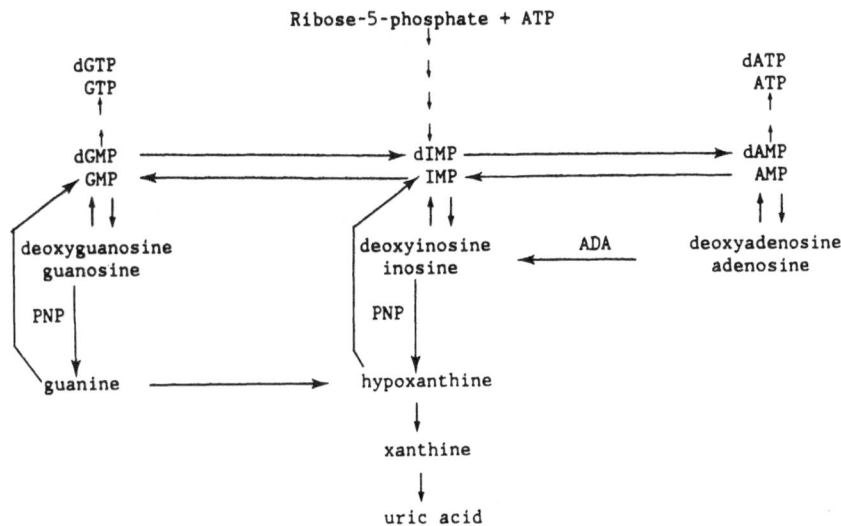

Figure 6.1 Purine metabolic pathway

Purine nucleoside phosphorylase (PNP; purine orthophosphate ribosyltranferase EC 2.4.2.1)

The enzyme, PNP, catalyses the conversion of inosine and deoxyinosine into hypoxanthine and of guanosine and deoxyguanosine into guanine (Figure 6.1). Like ADA, PNP is present in most body tissues, the highest activity being found in human erythrocytes. Peripheral blood T and B lymphocytes do not significantly differ in PNP activity. However, as compared to peripheral blood T cells, the activity in thymocytes is low. PNP has a molecular weight of 84 kDa, consisting of three identical 28 kDa subunits. Starch gel electrophoresis of red cell lysates shows several bands of PNP activity due to post-translational modification of the enzyme. Polymorphisms of PNP are not known[5, 7]. The PNP structural gene is located[18] on the long arm of chromosome 14.

Patients with PNP deficiency have absent or less than 0.5% enzyme activity. However, two brothers have been described with delayed onset selective cellular immune deficiency and residual erythrocyte PNP activity of about 0.5%[7]. The electrophoretic findings in haemolysates of the parents of PNP patients, which usually have about 50% of the normal enzyme activity, may vary since both normal and abnormal electrophoretic patterns have been found. The former pattern is usually associated with a lack of immunologically detectable inactive PNP protein, whereas in the latter inactive PNP protein is present. The abnormal electrophoretic pattern in the latter is due to the presence of heterodimers composed of normal and inactive PNP monomer subunits[5].

Metabolic abnormalities

Deficiency of ADA or PNP results in characteristic urinary excretion patterns of purine metabolites (Table 6.2). ADA deficient patients excrete large amounts of adenosine and deoxyadenosine[16], while PNP deficient patients excrete markedly elevated levels of guanosine, deoxyguanosine, inosine and deoxyinosine[4, 5]. Hypouricosuria is a feature of the latter[4]. The plasma of ADA and PNP deficient patients has a similar profile of metabolites to that of the urine, and these abnormalities are even detectable at birth in cord blood. As mentioned earlier, lymphocyte numbers and *in vitro* lymphocyte function at birth can be completely normal despite these metabolic abnormalities. As yet we have no satisfactory explanation for this.

Pathogenic mechanisms

The finding that two consecutively acting enzymes in the purine catabolic pathway are associated with two distinct immune deficiency syndromes raises some important questions on how purine enzymes may regulate lymphocyte function. Much research has been done in the past 10 years on this issue and a clearer picture is emerging. In ADA deficiency, the metabolite deoxyadenosine has a detrimental effect on the development and function of the lymphoid system, whereas in PNP deficiency deoxyguanosine is the culprit[5, 7].

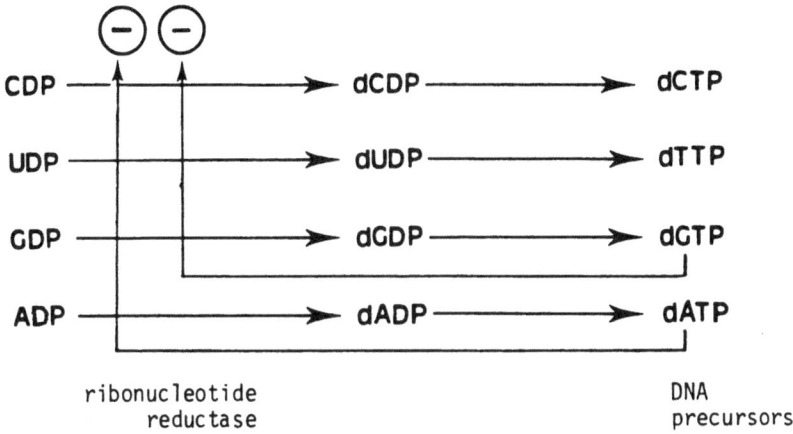

Figure 6.2 Feedback inhibition of ribonucleotide reductase by dATP and dGTP

These conclusions are derived from studies on either cells of the patients themselves or from studies performed in *in vitro* model systems for ADA or PNP deficiency. The former studies show that ADA deficient patients accumulate deoxyadenosine triphosphate (dATP) in their erythrocytes and lymphocytes[19]. In addition, the lymphocytes show increased concentrations of cyclic AMP (Table 6.2). In PNP deficient patients, high levels of deoxyguanosine triphosphate (dGTP) together with low levels of GTP are found in the erythrocytes[20]. Increased lymphocyte dGTP has been found in the few PNP deficient patients whose cells have been analysed (Table 6.2; ref. 14).

The model studies, discussed in more detail below, are in favour of the central mechanism being the accumulation of dATP or dGTP in lymphocytes which inhibits the enzyme, ribonucleotide reductase, which controls DNA synthesis and lymphocyte proliferation[5,7,21] (Figure 6.2). As far as ADA deficiency is concerned, recent findings on 'resting' lymphocytes show that deoxyadenosine is also toxic for non-dividing mature human T lymphocytes through a mechanism independent of inhibition of ribonucleotide reductase[22].

Table 6.2 Metabolic features of ADA and PNP deficiency

	ADA⁻	*PNP⁻*
Urine, plasma	adenosine↑ deoxyadenosine↑	inosine↑, deoxyinosine↑ guanosine↑, deoxyguanosine↑, uric acid↓
Erythrocytes	dATP↑	dGTP↑, GTP↓
Lymphocytes	dATP↑ cyclic AMP↑	dGTP↑

Furthermore, two additional mechanisms have been proposed for ADA deficiency: cyclic AMP-mediated modulation of immune function and Ado- and dAdo-mediated increase in S-adenosylhomocysteine, an inhibitor of methylation reactions, including methylation of DNA[16, 23]. Methylation reactions are required for a number of important cellular functions such as chemotaxis, cytotoxicity and capping and redistribution of membrane determinants.

EFFECTS OF dAdo AND dGuo IN MODEL SYSTEMS

Most model systems used to study the pathogenesis of PNP and ADA deficiency have been directed to the analysis of the toxic effects of accumulated substrates, and not the effect of a deficiency of metabolic products on the lymphoid system. This bias is understandable since deoxyguanosine, one of the accumulating substrates in PNP deficiency, was already known to inhibit DNA synthesis. The systems used included continuously growing mouse T cell lymphosarcoma (S49 cells) and human T-and B-lymphoblastoid cell lines with or without the enzyme deficiency. In addition, normal human peripheral blood T- and B lymphocytes stimulated with either mitogens or antigens in the presence of dAdo or dGuo have been used. As far as PNP deficiency is concerned, until recently no effective PNP inhibitor was available and the few *in vivo* studies consisted of injecting dGuo into experimental animals without inhibiting PNP. More recently the PNP inhibitor 8-NH$_2$ guanosine has become available.

Studies with dAdo

The fate of dAdo within a cell is primarily dependent on the activity of ADA by virtue of its low K_m of about $7\,\mu$mol/l. When ADA is deficient or inhibited (e.g. by deoxycoformycin) dAdo will be phosphorylated by deoxyadenosine kinase (K_m = $400\,\mu$mol/l) into dAMP, whereafter further phosphorylation into dADP and dATP takes place (Figure 6.3). In addition to the action of deoxyadenosine kinase, some workers have suggested that dAdo is phosphorylated by the enzyme deoxycytidine kinase[24, 25]. When cells from various sources were compared, it appeared that the highest activity of the deoxynucleoside kinases was found in thymocytes, followed by peripheral blood T cells. Contradictory results have been published on the activity of deoxynucleoside kinase in peripheral blood B cells, with both lower and equal activities of the enzymes being found to those in T cells[25].

The potential capacity of dAdo to inhibit cell growth can easily be demonstrated by either addition of dAdo to cultures of human peripheral blood T lymphocytes pretreated with deoxycoformycin and stimulated with mitogens, or to lymphoblastoid ADA deficient T and B cell lines. In the mouse T-lymphosarcoma (S49) cell system, it has been unequivocally demonstrated that under ADA deficient conditons, dAdo can only exert its growth inhibitory effect when it is transported into the cell and phosphorylated to accumulate as dATP. Studies on the ADA deficient lymphoblastoid cell lines show that, in general, human T lymphoblasts are

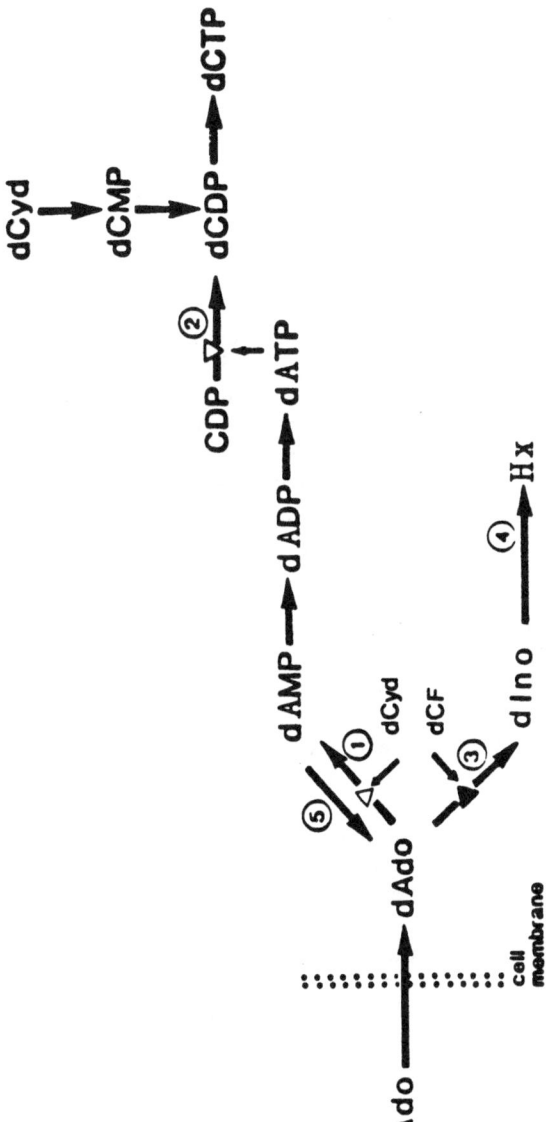

Figure 6.3 Intracellular pathways of deoxyadenosine. Enzymes: (1) deoxyadenosine kinase; (2) ribonucleotide reductase; (3) adenosine deaminase; (4) purine nucleoside phosphorylase; (5) 5' nucleotidase. Competitive inhibition (▷) of (1) by deoxycytidine (dCyd) and of (2) by dATP. Inactivation (▶) of (3) by deoxycoformycin (dCF)

more sensitive to dAdo inhibition than B lymphoblasts[5, 7, 26]. Moreover, the T cell lines accumulate higher concentrations of dATP, although exceptions have been found. The explanation for this differential sensitivity has been ascribed to differences in phosphorylating and dephosphorylating activities between T and B cells. Whereas T cells have higher phosphorylating activity than B cells, by virtue of the higher activity of deoxynucleoside kinase, B cells have a higher dephosphorylating activity manifested by the higher 5'-nucleotidase activity[27].

These studies leave unanswered the mechanism of dAdo- and dATP-mediated toxicity in ADA deficient lymphocytes. The most informative studies concerning this issue came from the effect of adding deoxycytidine (dCyd), together with dAdo, to cultures of either mitogen-activated (deoxycoformycin-treated) peripheral blood T lymphocytes or to ADA deficient lymphoblastoid T cell lines. In both instances dCyd reversed the dAdo inhibition. The mechanism for this reversal depends on dCyd competing with dAdo for phosphorylation by deoxynucleoside kinase, thus lowering the entrapment of dATP (see Figure 6.3). These observations led to the view that at least one mechanism of dAdo toxicity involves dATP-mediated inhibition of ribonucleotide reductase, with consequent failure to generate enough dCTP for lymphocyte DNA synthesis[5, 7].

Several observations in ADA⁻ patients can be adequately explained by this model. For example, the finding that T cells are more sensitive to dAdo than B cells *in vitro* explains the normal B cell numbers in most patients. Moreover, among cells of the T cell lineage, thymocytes are the most efficient at phosphorylating dAdo, suggesting that early T cell differentiation is most affected in ADA patients. The mechanism of inhibition of ribonucleotide reductase is similar in PNP deficiency (see later) but it is not clear why ADA deficiency is clinically more severe. Additional mechanisms have therefore been proposed.

One of the first observations which challenged the sole involvement of ribonucleotide reductase was the fact that in order to obtain inhibition of *in vitro* lymphocyte proliferation, dAdo had to be present during the first 24 hours of the culture. Furthermore, a block in the G0–G1 interphase is effected in cultures of deoxycoformycin treated peripheral blood T cells activated with mitogens. Moreover, low concentrations of dAdo, under ADA deficient conditions, interfere with early events of T cell activation such as ligand-mediated intracellular Ca^{2+} increase, expression of interleukin 2 receptors and production of interleukin 2. All these phenomena are independent of DNA synthesis. Of particular interest is the finding that in the presence of deoxycoformycin, dAdo is also toxic for non-stimulated and non-dividing 'resting' mature human T cells[22]. The toxicity of dAdo in this situation requires dATP formation and can be prevented by dCyd. However, the presumed mechanism is completely different from the ribonucleotide reductase model since cell death is associated with accumulation of single-strand breaks of DNA, a decrease in RNA synthesis, depletion of NAD and finally a profound and lethal drop in ATP pools[16, 22].

To complete the survey of mechanisms causing immunodeficiency in ADA deficiency, mention should be made of the toxic effect of both Ado and dAdo on the enzyme, S-adenosylhomocysteine hydrolase, which converts S-adenosylhomocysteine into adenosine and homocysteine[23]. This hydrolase is decreased in the erythrocytes of patients with ADA deficiency. This would theoretically lead to an accumulation of S-adenosylhomocysteine which is a potent competitive inhibitor of S-adenosylmethionine-mediated methylation reactions (see also p. 118). Finally Ado alone, under ADA deficient conditions, will be phosphorylated by adenosine kinase and lead to depletion of PP-ribose-P, thereby inhibiting *de novo* purine and pyrimidine biosynthesis[5, 7].

The severe metabolic consequences of ADA deficiency for lymphoid cells illustrated above would be expected to compromise immunity and predispose to life-threatening infections. The severity of the disease may well be the result of dAdo or Ado-mediated toxicity through several concurrently acting mechanisms. In this respect it can be added that early observations revealed an inhibitory effect of simulated ADA deficiency on the increase of acid phosphatase activity in monocytes *in vitro* which is normally apparent after incubation[28]. Although the functional relevance of this finding remains to be determined, macrophage involvement in ADA deficiency may be important and probably contributes to the clinical picture.

Studies with dGuo

The fate of dGuo in a cell is primarily determined by the activity of PNP, which has a relatively low K_m of $50 \mu mol/l$ (Figure 6.4). The enzyme deoxycytidine kinase (K_m $400 \mu mol/l$) may phosphorylate dGuo into dGMP, whereafter dGDP and dGTP formation takes place[24, 25]. A separate deoxyguanosine kinase has not yet been described. Only the deoxynucleoside kinase pathway is operative in PNP deficiency.

The addition of dGuo to continuously growing PNP deficient lymphoblastoid cell lines showed that human T cell lines were highly sensitive to dGuo inhibition, whereas human B cell lines were usually resistant[5, 7]. Similar to ADA⁻ deficient T cell lines, the addition of dCyd to PNP⁻ lines protects the cells from the toxic effects of dGuo by competing for phosphorylation by deoxycytidine kinase (Figure 6.4). The involvement of ribonucleotide reductase and the accumulation of intracellular dGTP in dGuo toxicity has been directly shown in a PNP deficient mutant mouse T cell lymphosarcoma cell line. One of these mutant cell lines was resistant to the effect of dGuo despite accumulating dGTP. This can be explained by the presence of an altered ribonucleotide reductase, resistant to feed back inhibition by dGTP, which was also a feature of these mutant cells[29].

Studies with normal peripheral blood T lymphocytes show that dGuo, in a dose-dependent pattern, inhibits mitogen or antigen-induced T cell proliferation[30]. The inhibition is associated with intracellular increases of both GTP and dGTP pools. This apparently simple model for PNP deficiency was soon complicated by the finding that Guo also inhibited *in vitro* T cell proliferation. Moreover, the *in vitro* proliferation and differentiation of human peripheral blood B lymphocytes cultured with T cell replacing factors is also inhibited by dGuo and Guo[31]. This caused some

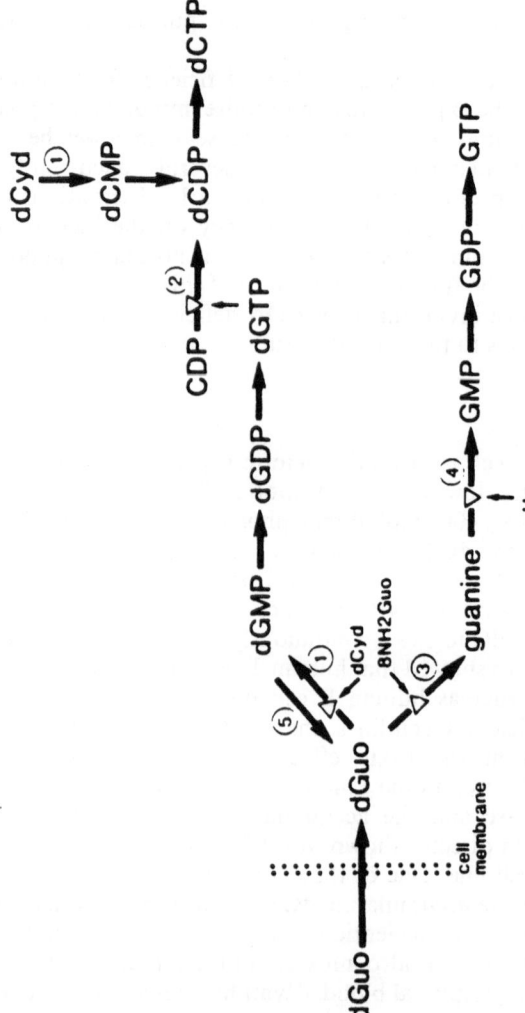

Figure 6.4 Intracellular pathways of deoxyguanosine. Enzymes: (1) deoxycytidine kinase; (2) ribonucleotide reductase; (3) purine nucleoside phosphorylase; (4) hypoxanthine–guanine phosphoribosyl transferase; (5) 5'-nucleotidase. Competitive inhibition ($\triangledown$) of (1) by deoxycytidine (dCyd), of (2) by dGTP and of (3) by 8NH$_2$guanosine (8NH$_2$Guo)

confusion since PNP deficient patients do have B cells which function normally. Analysis of the mechanism of dGuo and Guo toxicity in normal T and B cells showed the following results. The addition of dCyd only partially protected T cells from dGuo toxicity and there was no protection for B cells. Inhibition of PNP by $8NH_2$ guanosine, addition of hypoxanthine (competing with guanine for phosphorylation by HGPRT) and the use of HGPRT deficient lymphocytes from patients with the Lesch–Nyhan syndrome, lowered the toxicity of dGuo for T cells, and completely abrogated dGuo toxicity in B cells (see explanation in Figure 6.4). This clearly shows that there are two pathways of dGuo toxicity in normal T cells; namely the deoxycytidine kinase pathway and a pathway starting with dGuo (and Guo) degradation by PNP[30]. In normal B lymphocytes, only the latter is operative and the results with the HGPRT deficient cells indicate that the toxic product must be a compound beyond the enzyme HGPRT, i.e. GMP, GDP or GTP[31]. The message from these studies is that although the addition of dGuo to normal T cells mimics the functional effects of dGuo on PNP deficient T cells, the mechanism of dGuo toxicity in normal cells is not identical to the mechanism in PNP deficient cells.

It is apparent from the studies outlined above that purine nucleosides are potential regulators of normal T and B cell function. Moreover, we may conclude that B cells of PNP deficient patients are not sensitive to dGuo because the cells do not accumulate GMP, GDP and GTP, and therefore escape dGuo toxicity. Moreover B lymphocytes treated with dGuo in the presence of $8NH_2Guo$ do accumulate intracellular dGTP, however without any effect on B cell proliferation and differentiation[31].

It should be noted that T and B cells at different maturation stages may show a distinct susceptibility to dGuo. For instance, dGuo is very toxic to spontaneously proliferating immature CD3-negative thymocytes. The mechanism of this toxicity is similar to PNP deficient peripheral blood T cells, i.e. only the deoxycytidine kinase pathway is operative. The relatively high activity of deoxycytidine kinase and the very low activity of PNP in the $CD3^-$ thymocyte subset may account for this phenomenon. In contrast, more mature $CD3^+$ thymocytes have a similar sensitivity to dGuo toxicity as normal peripheral blood T lymphocytes. The extreme sensitivity of immature thymocytes to dGuo raises the question as to how some T cells of mature phenotype survive in PNP deficient patients. However, much of the T cell differentiation in the thymus of PNP deficient patients probably occurs in fetal or infant life, and it is possible that local dGuo concentrations are too low to affect differentiation at this stage. There is no information yet on the effect of dGuo and PNP deficiency on early B cell differentiation.

The abnormal metabolic findings in PNP deficient patients are generally in agreement with the results obtained in model systems. PNP deficiency is a syndrome where proliferation dependent functions of T lymphocytes are severely impaired, and the only mechanism so far demonstrated to account for this is ribonucleotide reductase inhibition by accumulated dGTP. T helper cell function, which, at least partially, is proliferation independent, is intact in these patients[4, 7]. In this context, it is interesting that autoimmune phenomena and 'autoimmune-like' diseases are common in PNP deficiency. Some authors relate this to defective suppressor T cell function which is dependent on lymphocyte proliferation[5, 7]. There are two pieces of evidence for defective T suppressor cell function in PNP deficiency: first, micromolar concentrations of dGuo interfere with the *in vitro* induction of antigen-specific suppressor cell function at the level of the precursor T suppressor-effector cell. Second, *in vivo* development of T suppressor-effector cells, operative in either antibody formation or in delayed-type hypersensitivity reactions in mice, can be abrogated by daily injections of dGuo. However, these studies have been done with normal PNP–containing cells. Although it is attractive to relate these findings to the occurrence of autoimmune phenomena in PNP deficient patients, definite proof is lacking, particularly since normal antigen specific T suppressor function has been demonstrated in a few PNP deficient patients.

THERAPY IN ADA AND PNP DEFICIENCY

Without treatment aimed to improve the immunological function, patients with ADA or PNP deficiency die of intractable infections during the first years of life. Several partially successful approaches to therapy are available. These comprise transplantation of lymphoid stem cells, enzyme replacement by way of repeated transfusions of irradiated erythrocytes, treatment with thymic humoral factors and deoxycytidine administration. Somatic gene therapy may soon be added to this list.

Bone marrow transplantation

Several ADA$^-$ SCID patients have been successfully treated with bone marrow from HLA identical donors, i.e. from matched siblings or phenotypically identical family members[16, 32]. Most of these resulted in immune reconstitution and no clinical signs of immune deficiency remained. The skeletal abnormalities usually also disappear after transplantation and in a few cases the neurological abnormalities have also improved. Engraftment of stem cells in ADA deficiency is accompanied by lowering of plasma and urine dAdo and Ado levels, the dATP levels in erythrocytes and lymphocytes also falling. However, these levels do not completely normalize, but are evidently low enough to enable *in vivo* differentiation of immunocompetent T and B cells[16]. It appears that bone marrow transplantation, apart from the delivery of stem cells, is also providing the machinery to clear dAdo. Interestingly, chimaeric states are often obtained after bone marrow transplantation of ADA deficient patients (i.e. a mixture of donor (ADA$^+$) and patient's (ADA$^-$) lymphocytes together with host (ADA$^-$) erythrocytes).

Unfortunately, no HLA identical siblings are available for some patients, and parental haploidentical bone marrow has been used with some temporary success. The final outcome for these patients is poor in contrast to the impressive results with other ADA$^+$ SCID infants. Results from both European and American centres for bone marrow transplantation show that transient engraftment associated with some improvement of lymphocyte function occurs in most patients, but is usually followed by loss of the graft and waning of immune function. One explanation for this failure is that donor stem cells or the T cells generated *in vivo* by thymus processing clear the toxic dAdo, which enables host stem cells to mature into T cells which reject the donor cells. In those patients who do not show any signs of engraftment the thymus microenvironment may be irreversibly damaged, precluding any T cell differentiation.

Experience with bone marrow transplantation is limited in PNP deficiency. Variable results have been obtained including engraftment and gradual immune reconstitution in one patient and loss of grafts or even no engraftment in others. The explanation for these poor results may be similar to that for ADA deficient patients. Thymus transplantation in a Dutch patient with PNP deficiency clinically induced healing of a generalized vaccinia infection and there was partial improvement of *in vitro* T cell function. However, the immunological benefit was transient, possibly because immunocompetent host T cells developed which rejected the thymus transplant. In this patient, a second and third thymus transplantation each effected transient partial improvement of *in vitro* T cell function.

Of particular clinical importance is the effect of bone marrow transplantation on the neurological abnormalities of PNP deficient patients. Although experience is very limited, this does not look promising.

Enzyme replacement

This is an alternative to bone marrow transplantation in ADA and PNP deficiency and can be achieved by repeated transfusions of irradiated ADA and PNP containing-erythrocytes from normal donors. It was shown as early as 1974 that this procedure may be beneficial to ADA⁻ SCID patients[33]. The donor red cells deaminate Ado and dAdo present in the body fluids and degrade them to purine bases and uric acid; Ado and dAdo levels in plasma and urine decrease and the dATP content of lymphocytes is lowered. However, only 50% of ADA⁻ SCID patients seem to respond clinically and immunologically to this procedure[5]. Actually, those patients having some residual immunological function before treatment do respond and those having no demonstrable T or B cell function do not, although the latter nevertheless display a decrease in toxic metabolites. This finding challenges the concept that clearing toxic metabolites is essential for successful treatment. However, the lack of response in these patients can be explained by either the loss of stem cells, pre-T cells and/or irreversible thymic damage from chronic exposure to toxic metabolites.

Experience with enzyme replacement by erythrocyte transfusions is limited to only a few patients with PNP deficiency. Long-term enzyme replacement for 6 years in a Dutch patient showed that 15 ml of irradiated packed red cells per kg bodyweight once a month maintained a low level of PNP activity in circulating erythrocytes. Each transfusion led to a decrease in nucleoside and deoxynucleoside excretion and a rise in uric acid. Enzyme replacement in this child partially corrected *in vitro* T cell function. However, lymphocyte counts remained very low and viral infections remained a problem.

Iron overload and transmission of hepatitis viruses are complications of regular erythrocyte transfusions. Moreover, permanent correction of T and B cell function has, to our knowledge, not been observed.

Thymic factors

The administration of thymic factors to patients with ADA or PNP deficiency could theoretically reverse the thymic deficiency, which may be responsible for failures with bone marrow transplantation or enzyme replacement by erythrocyte transfusions. However, thymic factors will only work if stem cells or pre-T cells are present, since it is these cells that have to be stimulated. One patient with ADA⁻ SCID did not improve on either enzyme replacement or thymosin alone, but immunological reconstitution and clinical improvement was achieved when both were combined.

Deoxycytidine administration

Based on insights into the mechanism(s) underlying defective lymphocyte differentiation and function in ADA and PNP deficiency, administration of deoxycytidine (dCyd) is theoretically a fourth therapeutic strategy (Figures 6.3 and 6.4). However, neither orally nor intravenously administered dCyd has benefited any patient. This is explained by degradation of the compound by cytidine deaminase in the gut mucosa and liver. It is possible to block this deaminase with tetrahydrouridine (THU), and experience in a Dutch patient showed that a regimen of 50 mg THU and 50 mg dCyd per kg bodyweight daily, both given subcutaneously, leads to detectable levels of dCyd in serum and urine, and more importanly to substantial levels of dCTP in the erythrocytes[34]. Unfortunately, the lymphocytes from this patient could not be investigated because of the severe lymphopenia. *In vitro* immune function, however, did not improve, possibly because of irreversible damage.

Somatic gene therapy

Recombinant DNA technology has led to the cloning of both the ADA and PNP gene. Furthermore, strategies have been developed for the introduction of foreign genetic material into somatic cells, including bone marrow stem cells, using retroviral vectors. Gene therapy for ADA and PNP deficiency is now in the realm of reality[35]. Both conditions seem suitable for gene therapy because it is technically feasible to obtain bone marrow precursor cells from the patients which can then be transfected with the genes. Furthermore, ADA and PNP are relatively simple enzymes coded by single genes, without complicated regulation of expression; partial correction of the enzyme deficiency may be enough to fully restore immune function.

CONCLUSIONS

The discovery of ADA and PNP deficiency has drawn attention to the intimate relationship between purine metabolism and lymphocyte differentiation. The apparently unique metabolism of dAdo and dGuo in thymocytes suggests an important role for deoxynucleosides in the physiology of intrathymic T cell differentiation, and it is possible that dGuo is responsible for the extensive cell death within the thymus which occurs during T cell differentiation. Measurements of local deoxynucleoside concentrations will be needed to prove a relationship.

The discovery of ADA deficiency and the unravelling of the mechanisms of dAdo toxicity led to the clinical use of deoxycoformycin, a potent inhibitor of ADA, in the treatment of leukaemias and lymphomas of the T cell lineage. The results show that pharmacological inhibition of ADA *in vivo* induces lysis of both malignant lymphoblasts and normal T cells. Although such therapy is highly effective in some patients who fail to respond to standard cytotoxic regimes, serious side-effects such as renal failure account for its diminishing popularity. Other anticancer drugs are known to have more or less selective effects on lymphocytes since they are phosphorylated by deoxycytidine kinase. These drugs include adenine-arabinoside, cytosine-arabinoside and guanine-arabinoside. However, malignant cells become resistant to these deoxynucleoside analogues by increasing their *de novo* synthesis of deoxynucleosides, including dCyd which competes with the drug for phosphorylation.

Despite important progress in understanding the metabolic consequences of ADA and PNP deficiency, the gradual involution of the immune system, the heterogeneity of clinical and immunological findings and the occurrence of autoimmune phenomena in PNP deficient patients, are not satisfactorily explained. It is important to make the diagnosis of ADA and PNP deficiency as early as possible to avoid irreversible damage of the lymphoid system, and possibly the central nervous system in the latter. Prenatal diagnosis is possible for both diseases, and somatic gene therapy will hopefully soon be available.

References

1. Giblett, E. R., Anderson, J. E., Cohen, F., Pollara, B. and Meuwissen, H. J. (1972). Adenosine deaminase deficiency in two patients with selectively impaired cellular immunity. *Lancet*, 2, 1067-9
2. Dissing, J. and Knudsen, J. B. (1972). Adenosine deaminase deficiency and combined immunodeficiency syndrome. *Lancet*, 2, 1316
3. Giblett, E. R., Ammann, A. J., Wara, D. W., Sandman, R. and Diamond, L. K. (1975). Nucleoside phosphorylase deficiency in a child with severely impaired cellular immunity. *Lancet*, 2, 1010-13
4. Stoop, J. W., Zegers, B. J. M., Hendrickx, G. F. M., Siegenbeek van Heukelom, L. H., Staal, G. E. J., de Bree, P. K., Wadman, S. K. and Ballieux, R. E. (1977). Purine nucleoside phosphorylase deficiency associated with selective cellular immunodeficiency. *N. Engl. J. Med.*, 296, 651-5
5. (1979). *Enzyme Defects and Immune Dysfunction*. Ciba Symp. 68, pp. 1-289. (Amsterdam, Oxford, New York: Excerpta Medica)
6. Hitzig, W. H., Döhmann, U., Plüss, H. J. and Vischer, D. (1974). Hereditary transcobalamine II deficiency: clinical findings in a new family. *J. Pediatr.*, 85, 622-8
7. Martin, D. W. and Gelfand, E. W. (1981). Biochemistry of diseases of immuno development. *Ann. Rev. Biochem.*, 50, 845-77
8. Girot, R., Hamet, M., Perignon, J. L., Guesnu, M., Fox, R. M., Cartier, P., Durandy, A. and Griscelli, C. (1983). Cellular immunodeficiency in two siblings with hereditary orotic aciduria. *N. Engl. J. Med.*, 308, 700-5
9. Cowan, M. J., Wara, D., Packman, S. and Ammann, A. J. (1979). Multiple biotine-

dependent carboxylase deficiencies associated with defects in T cell and B cell immunity. *Lancet*, **2**, 115-18

10. Bach, J. F. (1981). The multifaceted zinc dependency of the immune system. *Immunol. Today*, **2**, 225-7

11. Cohen, A., Mansour, A., Dosch, H. M. and Gelfand, E. W. (1980). Association of a lymphocyte purine enzyme deficiency (5' nucleotidase) with combined immunodeficiency. *Clin. Immunol. Immunopathol.*, **15**, 245-50

12. Watson, A. R., Evans, D. J. K., Marsden, N. B., Miller, V. and Rogers, P. A. (1981). Purine nucleoside phosphorylase deficiency associated with a fatal lymphoproliferative disorder. *Arch. Dis. Child.*, **56**, 563-5

13. Rÿksen, G., Kuis, W., Wadman, S. K., Spaapen, L. J. M., Duran, M., Voorbrood, B. S., Staal, G. E. J., Stoop J. W. and Zegers, B. J. M. (1987). A new case of purine nucleoside phosphorylase deficiency: enzymologic, clinical and immunological characteristics. *Pediatr. Res.*, **21**, 137-41

14. Simmonds, H. A., Watson, A. R., Webster, D. R., Sahoto, A. and Perrett, D. (1982). GTP depletion and other erythrocyte abnormalities in inherited PNP deficiency. *Biochem. Pharmacol.*, **31**, 941-6

15. Borkowsky, W., Gershon, A. A., Shenkman, L. and Hirschhorn, R. (1988). Adenosine deaminase deficiency without immunodeficiency: clinical and metabolic studies. *Pediatr. Res.*, **14**, 885-9

16. (1985). Adenosine deaminase in disorders of purine metabolism and in immune deficiency. *Ann. N. Y. Acad. Sci.*, **451**, 1-342

17. Creagan, R. P., Tischfield, J. A., Nichols, E. A. and Ruddle, F. H. (1973). Autosomal assignment of the gene for adenosine deaminase which is deficient in patients with combined immunodeficiency syndrome. *Lancet*, **2**, 1449-51

18. Franke, U., Busby, N., Shaw, D., Hansen, S. and Bronn, M. G. (1976). Intrachromosomal gene mapping in man: assignment of nucleoside phosphorylase to region 14 cen → 14q21 by intraspecific hybridization of cells with a t(x:14) (p22:q21) translocation. *Som. Cell Genet.*, **2**, 27-40

19. Cohen, A., Hirschhorn, R., Horowitz, S. D., Rubinstein, A., Polmar, S. H., Hong, R. and Martin, D. W. Jr. (1978). Deoxyadenosine triphosphate as a potentially toxic metabolite in adenosine deaminase deficiency. *Proc. Natl. Acad. Sci. USA*, **75**, 472-6

20. Cohen, A., Gudas, L. J., Ammann, A. J., Staal, G. E. J. and Martin, D. W. Jr. (1978). Deoxyguanosine triphosphate as a possible toxic metabolite in the immunodeficiency associated with purine nucleoside phosphorylase deficiency. *J. Clin. Invest.*, **61**, 1404-9

21. Reichard, P. (1978). From deoxynucleotides to DNA synthesis. *Fed. Proc.* **37**, 9-13

22. Seto, S., Carrera, C. J., Wasson, D. B. and Carson, D. A. (1984). Mechanism of deoxyadenosine and 2-chlorodeoxyadenosine toxicity to non-dividing human lymphoyctes. *J. Clin. Invest.*, **75**, 377-88

23. Hershfield, M. S. (1979). Apparent suicide inactivation of human lymphoblast S-adenosylhomocysteine hydrolase by 2'-deoxyadenosine and adenine arabinoside: a basis for direct toxic effects of analogs of adenosine. *J. Biol. Chem.*, **254**, 22-4

24. Carson, D. A., Kaye, J. and Seegmiller, J. E. (1977). Lymphospecific toxicity in adenosine deaminase deficiency and purine nucleoside phosphorylase deficiency: possible role of nucleoside kinase(s). *Proc. Natl. Acad. Sci. USA*, **74**, 5677-81

25. Osborne, W. A. (1986). Nucleoside kinases in T and B lymphoblasts distinguished by autoradiography. *Proc. Natl. Acad. Sci. USA*, **83**, 4030-4

26. Mitchell, B. S., Mejias, E., Daddona, P. E. and Kelley, W. N. (1978). Purinogenic immunodeficiency diseases: selective toxicity of deoxyribonucleosides for T cells. *Proc. Natl. Acad. Sci. USA*, **75**, 5011-14

27. Carson, D. A., Wasson, D. B., Lakow, E. and Katamani, N. (1982). Possible metabolic basis for the different immunodeficiency states associated with genetic deficiencies of adenosine deaminase and purine nucleoside phosphorylase. *Proc. Natl. Acad. Sci. USA*, **79**, 3848-52

28. Fischer, D., van der Weyden, M. B., Snijderman, R. and Kelley, W. N. (1976). A role for adenosine deaminase in human monocyte maturation. *J. Clin. Invest.*, **58**, 399-407

29. Ullman, B., Gudas, L. J., Clift, S. M. and Martin, D. W. Jr. (1979). Isolation and characterization of purine nucleoside phosphorylase deficient T lymphoma cells and secondary mutants with altered ribonucleotide reductase: genetic model for immunodeficiency disease. *Proc. Natl. Acad. Sci. USA*, **76**, 1074-8

30. Spaapen, L. J., Rijkers, G. T., Staal, G. E. J., Rijksen, G., Wadman, S. K., Stoop, J. W. and Zegers, B. J. M. (1984). The effect of deoxyguanosine on human lymphocyte function. I. Analysis of the interference with lymphocyte proliferation. *J. Immunol.*, **132**, 2311-17
31. Scharenberg, J. G. M., Spaapen, L. J., Rijkers, G. T., Duran, M., Staal, G. E. J. and Zegers, B. J. M. (1986). Functional and mechanistic studies on the toxicity of deoxyguanosine for the *in vitro* proliferation and differentiation of human peripheral blood B lymphocytes. *Eur. J. Immunol.*, **16**, 381-7
32. Hirschorn, R. (1980). Treatment of genetic diseases by allotransplantation. In Desnick, R. J. (ed.) *Birth Defects*. Original Article Series. Vol. 16, no. 1, pp. 429-44. March of Dimes
33. Polmar, S. H., Stern, R. C., Schwartz, A. L., Wetzer, E. M., Chase, P. A. and Hirschhorn, R. (1976). Restoration of *in vitro* lymphocyte responses with exogenous adenosine deaminase in a patient with severe combined immunodeficiency. *N. Engl. J. Med.*, **195**, 1337-43
34. Rijkers, G. T., Zegers, B. J. M., Spaapen, L. J. M., Rutgers, D. H., Roord, J. J., Kuis, W. and Stoop, J. W. (1986). Purine nucleoside phosphorylase deficiency leading to accumulation of lymphocytes in S-phase. *Pediatr. Hemat. Oncol.*, **3**, 353-9
35. Williams, D. A. and Orkin, S. H. (1985). Somatic gene therapy: current status and future prospects. *J. Clin. Invest.*, **77**, 1053-6

7
Interferon Deficiency Syndrome

S. LEVIN

HISTORICAL

Although the classic publications of Isaacs and Lindenmann in 1957 were the first to introduce the term interferon (IFN) to the nomenclature of biology[1], much related important and interesting research over a period of 15 years preceded their report in which a viral-growth-interfering substance was described which was produced and secreted by cells infected by viruses[2]. Their discovery was that this substance, present in supernatants from virus-infected allantoic cells, prevented further viral replication when added to newly-infected cell cultures. Subsequently, it was shown that although there were numerous inducers of IFN production by cells, viruses were the most potent and that all viruses have this IFN-stimulating potential. Moreover, double-stranded RNA was the key to the induction of IFN. However, non-viral induction of IFN was also reported, usually to a much lesser degree, and these inducers included endotoxins, bacteria, synthetic polyanions and plant lectins[3].

It soon became apparent that there were several types of IFN produced by different cells with differences in their molecular structure and biological properties. To date, three main classes of IFN have been described in man: IFN-α, IFN-β and IFN-γ, with several subclasses of IFN-α and possibly of the others also. Viruses induce mainly IFN-α production by cells, whereas phytohaemagglutinin (PHA), concanavalin-A (Con-A), other mitogens and some antigens give rise to 'immune' IFN or IFN-γ production by T lymphocytes. IFN-β is produced by fibroblasts stimulated by viruses. The advent of genetically-engineered recombinant interferons (rIFN) has led to the synthesis in large amounts of the classic IFNs as well as numerous novel subclasses of IFNs, so far mainly of IFN-α. Because of the vast amount of research performed on this exciting new natural antiviral substance over the years, it soon became ovbious that the IFNs had several other biological activities of which modulation of the immune system and retardation of cell growth were the most obvious. Because of this, the clinical use of IFN in the treatment of neoplastic disease soon outweighed its use as an antiviral agent.

INTERFERON ACTIONS

Antiviral effect

Although it is over 25 years since the original description of the antiviral effect of IFN, only now are we beginning to understand its mode of action and its role in human biology. It seems that the IFN system is relatively dormant when an individual is healthy, and is activated only when cells are stimulated by viruses, mitogens, antigens, microbials and other inducers. This system consists of circulating white blood cells as well as cells of different organs and tissues which are potential sources of IFN production, together with the target cells which respond to IFN stimulation. The antiviral action is a two-stage mechanism in which entry of virus into a cell triggers the production of molecules of IFN, which are secreted from the cell into the surrounding tissue fluids. The second stage begins when the IFN molecules react with an IFN receptor on a cell-membrane (IFN-α and IFN-β have a common receptor whilst IFN-γ has its own receptor), thereby setting in motion a series of intracellular events leading to the activation of at least three antiviral enzymes whose functions are to prevent viral recognition, translation of viral RNA and assembly of new virus should another virus enter the cell[3]. This activated cell is then in an antiviral state and further viral replication is inhibited or markedly diminished, depending on the proportion of cells converted into an antiviral state.

It is known that IFN levels in the blood may become elevated within hours of the occurrence of viraemia, suggesting the importance of IFN in the early immune response against viruses. Our experience suggests that the antiviral state of cells, as established by studies on peripheral blood mononuclear cells (PBMC), is induced within 24–48 hours following appearance of IFN in the blood, and may persist for several days after IFN levels (the half-life of IFN is about 4 hours) have dropped and become non-assayable[4]. It has also been shown by us and others that simultaneous *in vivo* production of mixtures of HuIFN-α with either HuIFN-β or HuIFN-γ do occur, and it is believed that different proportions or combinations of interferons may have different specific cell effects.

Anti-cell-growth effect

The mechanism whereby the IFNs inhibit or slow down cell proliferation and differentiation is as yet purely speculative. Interference by IFN of intracellular protein synthesis has been suggested by some authors, and others have speculated that changes induced in cell membranes are responsible for this effect. Some have been tempted to speculate that IFN may act to control gene expression by some action at the level of transcription[5]. However, what has been proposed so far does not adequately explain the IFN effect on cell growth.

Immune function regulation

Immune modulation is an important function of the IFNs which act as biological messengers communicating between various cells of the immune system as well as with cells of other systems. It has been shown that the primary function of IFN-γ, which is produced by T cells following antigen stimulation, is immunoregulatory, although it does have some antiviral activity like IFN-α and IFN-β. Many other substances besides the IFNs can influence the immune system, but the direct effect of IFN on B cells, T cells, killer cells and macrophages has been proven beyond doubt[6]. It appears that there are selective effects of the different IFNs on various cells; conversely different target cells, including tumour cell lines, respond differently to the various IFNs. Of interest, and as yet unexplained, is that in certain instances IFN may act as an immune stimulant, and at other times as an immune suppressant; this is sometimes related to a dose-effect. It has been suggested that the appearance of an unusual IFN-α which is pH2-labile – unlike the classic IFN-α, in the serum of patients with systemic lupus erythematosus or AIDS and which may persist for long periods, may contribute to the dysfunction of the immune system in these disorders[6]. It is apparent that in many ways this 'immune' IFN-γ is different from the other IFNs, not only by having a different receptor to the common one for IFN-α and IFN-β, but also because its gene, which has three introns, is located on chromosome 12, whilst the genes for the other two, which have no introns, are found on chromosome 3.

ACTIVATION OF THE INTERFERON SYSTEM

The production of IFN and its appearance in the circulation is an important and early defence mechanism against viral infections. A competent IFN response, which includes induction of an antiviral state in cells and stimulation of numerous immune defence activities, is probably the major mechanism for limiting most viral infections to a few days of symptomatology followed by a complete and rapid recovery. Certainly this quick response helps in controlling the spread of infection until other slower-developing immune mechanisms can operate. Undoubtedly, this is not the entire picture, as we know that in some acute and many chronic viral infections, viral replication and spread occur despite an activated IFN system; the reason for this is not clear.

DEFECTIVE INTERFERON RESPONSE RESULTS

Deficiencies of immune mechanisms related to the lymphocyte, granulocyte and complement systems have been well described[7], and we have previously reported 15 cases with markedly defective IFN responses to an acute viral infection[8]. In this review we report an additional three cases of this IFN deficiency syndrome which is characterized by absent *in vivo* IFN production, inability of the patient's peripheral blood mononuclear cells (PBMC) to produce IFN-α and IFN-γ *in vitro*, and PBMC which were not in an antiviral state at the height of an acute viral infection. Of 18 patients diagnosed as having this deficiency syndrome only one had assayable IFN in the blood and another single patient had PBMC in an antiviral state. Eleven failed to

Table 7.1 18 patients with IFN deficiency syndrome

| Patient | Diagnosis | (Age) | Outcome | IFN production (units/ml) | | | Antiviral state of PBMC* |
| | | | | In vivo | In vitro | | |
				Serum IFN	IFN-α	IFN-γ	
	Normal healthy persons (n=75)			5±1.4†	382±62	170±26	(10^5)
	Acute viral infections (n=291)			76±9.7	215±14	165±15	$+(10^2)$
1.	Herpes fulminant hepatitis	(18 months)	#D	0	0	0	$-(10^5)$
2.	Fulminant hepatitis A	(47 years)	#R	0	0	0	$-(10^7)$
3.	Fulminant hepatitis + malnutrition	(4 months)	D	0	0	0	$-(10^4)$
4.	Fulminant hepatitis non-A non-B	(6 years)	D	0	0	0	$-(10^4)$
5.	Herpes simplex + pyoderma gangrenosum	(36 years)	#R	0	0	0	$-(10^7)$
6.	Herpes simplex + Hodgkin's	(40 years)	#R	0	0	0	$-(10^4)$
7.	Herpes encephalitis	(4 months)	D	0	0	0	$-(10^4)$
8.	Herpes encephalitis	(18 years)	D	0	0	0	$-(10^4)$
9.	Herpes encephalitis	(24 years)	D	0	0	0	$-(10^5)$
10.	Fulminant hepatitis A + pregnancy	(20 years)	#D	0	0	0	$-(10^5)$
11.	Toxic varicella (post measles)	(15 months)	#R	0	0	0	$-(10^7)$
12.	Progressive hepatitis A	(4 years)	#R	0	8	27	$-(10^3)$
13.	Fulminant hepatitis non-A non-B	(11 years)	#R	0	32	0	$-(10^7)$
14.	Fulminant hepatitis B	(66 years)	#D	0	64	0	$-(10^7)$
15.	Fulminant hepatitis B	(23 years)	#R	0	125	0	$-(10^5)$
16.	AIDS (terminal)	(28 years)	D	0	0	5	$+(10^0)$
17.	AIDS (terminal)	30 years)	D	0	4	18	$-(10^5)$
18.	Measles (severe), pneumothorax	(1½ years)	#D	4	0	0	ND

*Antiviral state is present when <10^3 virus is found after 48 hours culture of 10^3 TCID$_{50}$ VSV on PBMC; (+ = present, - = absent).
#=treated; R=recovered; D=died; n=number; †mean±1SE; PBMC=peripheral blood mononuclear cells

produce IFN-α or IFN-γ *in vitro* and the remaining seven could produce only minimal amounts (Table 7.1). The methods used in these assays have been previously described in detail[9]. In an assay used to determine whether the patient's intrinsic intracellular antiviral mechanism was competent, addition of small amounts (from 8 to 64 units) of IFN-α *in vitro* to the assay system led to induction of an antiviral state in the PBMC of all patients, suggesting that the primary cause of the lack of development of an antiviral state of cells was the absence of IFN rather than a defective intracellular mechanism. As expected, patients with this deficiency failed to control their viral infections which spread, and led invariably to death unless exogenous IFN-α was given as specific treatment. This exogenous IFN stopped the progressive deterioration in the patient's condition, stimulated *in vivo* IFN production, activated IFN-dependent immune mechanisms, induced an antiviral state in PBMC and led to recovery in seven out of 11 patients. In general, we found that in most cases an antiviral state of PBMC cells was induced within 1–3 days following onset of IFN-α therapy, and clinical improvement was noted within 4–5 days. In several cases the IFN response returned quite rapidly to normal as evidenced by the ability of PBMC to once again produce IFN-α and IFN-γ on appropriate *in vitro* stimulation[8]. Seven patients who did not receive IFN therapy died. All the evidence in these cases, who were mainly adults or older children who had not apparently had previous serious viral illness, suggests that this defective IFN response was acquired transiently, and was related to overwhelming viral infection which is known to suppress some immune responses[10]. The fact that nine of the 18 cases were due to hepatitis viruses (HA, HB and non-A non-B), five due to herpes infections, two to measles and two to HIV (AIDS), suggests a possible direct suppressive effect of these viruses on the IFN-producing system[10]. There is no evidence as yet, however, of a virus that specifically inhibits *in vitro* IFN production in cell lines.

The following five case reports illustrate a successful outcome after HuIFN-α therapy (numbered as in Table 7.1).

Case 2 A 47-year-old man with rapid-onset acute liver failure developed grade 4 coma due to HAV. A dramatic clinical improvement occurred on the fifth day of HuIFN-α therapy, coinciding with activation of the IFN system which previously had been completely deficient. The patient also had renal failure with sepsis, which were successfully treated. Recovery from hepatitis was complete.

Case 5 A 35-year-old man with acute myeloblastic leukaemia developed a progressive, extensive gangrenous herpes simplex infection of the abdominal wall following appendectomy. He was critically ill, severely toxic, and had no *in vivo* or *in vitro* IFN responses. After 1 day of HuIFN-α therapy the patient's cells entered into an antiviral state. The infection was brought under control after 2 days of therapy, and subsequent recovery was rapid.

Case 6 A 40-year-old man with Hodgkin's disease developed a rapidly spreading herpes simplex infection of the skin. There was dramatic clinical improvement after 2 days of HuIFN-α therapy and rapid recovery thereafter.

This was the only case in which the patient's IFN system showed no response even after 5 days of therapy.

Case 12 A 4-year-old girl who had suffered for 6 weeks from progressive jaundice due to HAV developed grade 2-3 coma and became progressively drowsy and unresponsive. 4 days after starting HuIFN-α therapy the IFN system was activated, an antiviral state of cells developed and *in vitro* IFN-α and IFN-γ production were observed. At the same time she showed dramatic clinical and biochemical improvement and thereafter recovered rapidly.

Case 15 A 23-year-old woman in the 6th month of pregnancy progressed rapidly into terminal grade 4 coma 5 days after the onset of jaundice due to hepatitis B. After 4 days of HuIFN-α injections the patient recovered consciousness, and within a further week was ambulatory. Prior to therapy the *in vivo* IFN system was completely defective and there was no IFN production *in vitro*. 2 days after starting treatment the patient's cells were in an antiviral state and there was evidence of IFN production *in vitro*. She recovered fully, and subsequently gave birth to a normal infant with no evidence of disease.

THE INTERFERON SYSTEM IN HEALTH AND DISEASE

Since 1978 we have performed a battery of laboratory assays developed to evaluate the IFN system response to disease in over 2600 persons, including healthy individuals and patients suffering from a variety of diseases[4]. The blood of healthy individuals contains virtually no IFN, their PBMC are not normally in an antiviral state, but their PBMC are capable of responding *in vitro* to appropriate stimuli by producing both IFN-α and IFN-γ[4]. In acute viral infections blood IFN levels are significantly increased, and an antiviral state, defined as the inability of virus to replicate in the patient's PBMC in culture, is found in at least 2/3 of cases[4] (Table 7.1). The importance of the IFN response in viral illnesses is indicated by the increased amounts of IFN found in the blood within hours of the appearance of viraemia and the early activation of IFN-dependent secondary immune responses[11]. Increased natural killer activity, for example, may be induced *in vitro* within an hour after adding IFN to the cells[11]. In some patients with viral illness no detectable IFN was found in the blood in spite of being in the acute viraemic phase. One possible reason for this is that blood IFN levels are known to fluctuate, partly on account of the very short half-life (+ 4 hours) of circulating IFN. Another possibility is that the infecting virus in these cases might be a poor interferonogen, as has been observed, for example, in patients with respiratory syncytial virus infections[12]. The hypothesis that massive viraemia may interfere with IFN production has not been proved. We also found patients who were in an acute phase of viral disease with relatively low IFN blood levels (8-32 units/ml) and in whom an antiviral state was absent. This could be explained by the great variability which we found in the amount of added IFN needed (ranging from 8 to 128 units/ml) to induce an antiviral state *in vitro*. In some cancer patients this relative resistance to the induction of an antiviral state is relatively pronounced[13]. Our own studies have demonstrated the induction of an antiviral state in PBMC following intramuscular injections of IFN within 24 hours in some cases, and in other cases only after 3–4 days or longer. The reasons for the variability in the time factor are unclear although one possible explanation could be individual differences in sensitivity of PBMC to IFN induction of an antiviral state. Another possibility may be related to the class or combination of classes of IFN produced and present in the blood, each having different capabilities for inducing the antiviral state. Other theoretical possibilities implicate defective intracellular antiviral mechanisms (for example, deficient production of antiviral enzymes), or IFN receptor defects on cell membranes. Once an antiviral state has been induced in PBMC it tends to persist for several days after IFN levels have become undetectable. Amongst the patients studied we found several whose PBMC did not produce either IFN-α or IFN-γ following *in vitro* stimulation with poly-IC or PHA respectively. However, absence of both IFN-α and IFN-γ production in the same patient is unusual and has only been seen in a few of our cases.

If the speed of the IFN response to viral infection is important, delay in producing endogenous IFN (or an inability to produce it) may lead to uninhibited progression of the viral infection. All the sick patients with undetectable blood IFN, absent antiviral state and defective or absent IFN production by PBMC *in vitro* shared a common feature; they all had progressive viral disease leading to severe or prolonged illness and in some cases death. It should be noted that not all critically ill patients with acute unresponsive viral illnesses had defective IFN responses as measured by our assay systems, and thus the reason for progressive infection in these latter patients must be sought elsewhere. As we have previously shown, the intracellular IFN antiviral mechanism was intact in all our patients as indicated by the ability to induce an antiviral state in their PBMC *in vitro* by the addition of 8–64 units/ml of IFN[8]. Thus the primary defect is an inability to produce endogenous IFN on appropriate stimulation.

RESPONSE TO IFN TREATMENT

Since it takes 4–5 days to complete the biological assays required to determine the integrity of the IFN system in any given patient, treatment with HuIFN-α in the most severely ill patients was usually started before the results were known. In patients whose intracellular IFN system was subsequently found to be defective, but in whom an antiviral state was found to be inducible *in vitro*, IFN administration was associated in almost every case with *in vivo* induction of an antiviral state in the cells. Daily monitoring showed that in one case the antiviral state was induced within 24 hours of injecting IFN, in others it took 2–5 days to develop, and in one case was not detected at all until recovery. In some patients *in vitro* IFN-α or IFN-γ production became evident within 1–10 days of starting IFN therapy. In patients who made complete recoveries, the IFN responses returned to normal, arguing against this deficiency being primary. In two critically ill patients with fulminant hepatitis, the IFN system was rapidly activated and *in vitro* IFN-α and IFN-γ production started almost immediately after commencing therapy. However, both patients died a few days later of extensive and irreversible tissue and organ damage. In patients who recovered clinical improvement was often observed to begin at approximately the time that an antiviral state was induced in their cells.

DEFECTIVE INTERFERON RESPONSES – REPORTS FROM THE LITERATURE

When we first described an IFN deficiency syndrome in 1980[14], there were several reports in the literature describing partial IFN system deficiencies in patients with viral infections or other diseases in which either *in vivo* or *in vitro* IFN-α or IFN-γ production was assayed and found defective. However, more extensive assays as described in the present report were not performed. Isaacs and co-workers reported deficient production of IFN-α by lymphocytes *in vitro* and in the nasal secretions *in vivo* in four young children with recurrent upper and lower rhinovirus respiratory tract infections[15]. In each case IFN-γ production by PBMC *in vitro* was normal. In three of the children repeated assays of *in vitro* IFN-α production remained negative over a period of a year and in the fourth patient IFN-α production was detected after 1 year, and later, two others began producing IFN-α. Only in one patient did the authors repeatedly fail to find IFN-α in the nasal secretions at the time of rhinovirus infection. Control patients with identical clinical and virological findings produced IFN-α normally both *in vivo* and *in vitro*. The possibility was raised that this was a primary defect which was genetically determined, because defective IFN-α production by lymphocytes was also found in two siblings of deficient producers (but not in the parents). This report therefore describes a partial IFN-α system deficiency, consisting of a transient IFN-α deficiency accompanied by recurrent viral respiratory infections in children.

Other than this isolated description of a possible primary defect of IFN-α production, all other reported instances of defective IFN production appear to be secondary to the effect of various disease processes on lymphocyte and leukocyte function. However, in a recent study in AIDS patients it was shown that *in vitro* IFN-γ production by PBMC stimulated with Con-A was normal despite a drastic decrease in T-helper cells. However, there was an impairment of IFN-γ production in response to specific antigens in these cases[16]. In most reports a single parameter was studied and usually not repeated. In some cases where IFN-α or IFN-γ production was found to be deficient, the second class of IFN was produced normally. In a few reports IFN production to a particular inducer was found to be defective, whilst the same IFN class was produced by PBMC with another stimulant. One must question whether these are true cases of IFN deficiency states or due to partial suppression of IFN production whose clinical significance is not apparent.

Virelizier and Griscelli described a 4-year-old boy with recurrent bacterial and viral infections in whom *in vitro* IFN production was consistently absent and natural killer cytotoxic activity was profoundly impaired[17]. Treatment with IFN reversed the natural killer defect, and this was accompanied by clinical improvement. In another report these same authors describe a 5-year-old girl with severe, persistent EBV infection in whom they could not find any detectable defect in humoral or cellular immunity except for a repeatedly observed selective defect of IFN-γ production by the PBMC[18]. The patient's *in vivo* IFN-α production was normal. In a third report they describe four patients with 'non-classical' cellular immune deficiencies in whom combined defects of IFN production and low natural killer activity were observed[19].

In a 1982 review a list of conditions in which a deficiency of either IFN-α or IFN-γ production had been described included normal newborns, congenital viral infections, Down's syndrome, certain primary immune deficiencies, and secondary immune deficiencies such as those found in uraemia, malnutrition and chronic hepatitis, as well as in patients on immunosuppressive therapy and/or, lymphatic malignancies[20]. Many of the studies cited in the review were again based on a single assay, and in none were attempts made to include more comprehensive evaluations of the IFN system. We, on the other hand, found normal or near normal *in vitro* IFN responses in newborn infants following PBMC stimulation with PHA and Poly-IC[21], while others have reported profound defects of IFN-γ production induced by PHA but normal production of IFN-α induced by Newcastle disease virus (NDV)[22]. It appears that the defective IFN-γ production in newborns could be due to the excessive suppressive effect of prostaglandin-E$_2$ on IFN-γ production and that this effect can be reversed by indomethacin[23].

At the opposite end of the spectrum, it was found that elderly persons had a significant decrease of IFN production *in vitro* to varicella zoster and herpes simplex antigens[24]. Our own study of elderly persons over the age of 75 years indicated that they had normal IFN responses (unpublished).

There appears to be no direct correlation between defects of the humoral or cellular immune systems and those of the IFN system. In some cases of IgA deficiency a defective T cell IFN response has been found, but in other B or T system immunodeficient patients no IFN defects were observed[25]. Normal IFN responses have been found in patients with thymic dysplasia[26] and with ataxia-telangiectasia[27]. More recently it was reported from Rome that *in vitro* IFN-γ production was abnormally low or undetectable in patients with ataxia-telangiectasia, combined immune deficiency, hyper-IgE syndrome and AIDS, but not in other immune deficiencies[28]. In most of these conditions there is a marked deficiency of T cells. In patients with Down's syndrome, in which there is evidence of a T cell defect, we found diminished IFN-α and IFN-γ production *in vitro*[29], although others found normal production[30]. The *in vivo* IFN response has been shown to be relatively resistant to immunosuppression by drugs, irradiation or anti-lymphocyte serum[20], although a recent report on cyclosporin-treated and conventionally immunosuppressed patients showed that in some cases there was mild impairment of IFN-α and IL-2 production, but there was no effect of cyclosporin on *in vitro* IFN-α production[31]. Our own studies have not shown any significant suppression of the IFN response in patients receiving steroids, and recently it was reported that steroids did not influence *in vitro* IFN-α production[32], and apparently may even augment release of IFN-α in virus-stimulated human lymphoid cell lines[33].

Other than in selected cases of hepatitis virus, herpes and measles infections in our own studies, defective or deficient IFN production has been reported with a few other viral infections. As early as 1974 it was found that infants suffering from symptomatic congenital cytomegalovirus (CMV) infections had defective IFN-α production when compared to non-symptomatic CMV carriers[34]. We now know that this is associated with an underlying primary or secondary immune deficiency in most, if not all, cases. Treatment of these CMV-infected patients with IFN-α has not proven satisfactory. Some cases of Reye's syndrome associated with influenzae B infections were shown to have defective *in vitro* INF-α production by their PBMC during the acute stage of the disease, but not during convalescence[35]. About 30% of persons with frequent episodes of herpes labialis are deficient in the production of herpes simplex virus-induced, immune specific IFN[36]. An unusual group of children suffering from recurrent respiratory tract and/or middle ear infections accompanied by arthralgias were found to have defective production of an atypical IFN-α (pH2-labile) which is probably produced by a subset of T lymphocytes when stimulated with *Staph. aureus* Cowan 1, but their responses to other inducers were normal[37]. In certain bacterial infections, such as tuberculosis, some patients were found to have defective IFN-γ production[38].

In recent years the association of the human immune deficiency virus (HIV) with AIDS has given rise to increased interest in the role of IFN in the development of this usually progressive viral disease. A study of *in vitro* lymphokine production in patients with AIDS showed deficient production of IFN-γ by PBMC induced with mitogens or specific microbial antigens[16]. Of interest was the finding that the addition of IFN-γ reversed abnormal monocyte function, suggesting a role for IFN in the treatment of this condition during opportunistic infections[16]. In African AIDS, IFN-α production by PBMC stimulated with Newcastle disease virus, as well as IFN-γ production, were found to be markedly defective, and there was a high correlation between the presence of circulating IFN and decreased IFN-γ production[39]. AIDS patients were also found to have diminished IFN responses to three viruses, CMV, HSV1 and HSV2[40]. We studied the IFN responses in a large cohort of clinically healthy homosexuals who were at risk for AIDS. About one-third of them had highly activated IFN responses when first examined. Blood IFN levels (mainly PH2-sensitive IFN-α) were exceedingly high, in some cases being >1000 units/ml, and IFN-α and IFN-γ production *in vitro* were often several times greater than in normal controls. Spontaneous IFN production too was markedly increased in these individuals, and 96% of them had PBMC in an antiviral state[9]. These findings suggested a continuing stimulation of the IFN system by viruses, and the increased unstimulated IFN production *in vitro* suggested the presence of intracellular virus or viral genome, as was later confirmed. What was remarkable was the fact that two of these individuals with the most highly activated IFN systems developed AIDS within 18 months, and terminally their IFN systems became deficient[9].

The situation with hepatitis viruses appears to be special. Our studies have shown that in certain rare cases of hepatitis virus infection, whether it be caused by HAV, HBV, herpes or non-A non-B viruses, there is a severe deficiency of the IFN response associated with a progressive and often fulminant illness. The *in vivo* and *in vitro* IFN values are significantly lower in fulminant hepatitis than in cases of hepatitis that run a normal course, and in most cases, IFN-α and IFN-γ production is zero on repeated testing[41]. All patients with fulminant hepatitis who did not receive HuIFN-α treatment died, whereas 75% of those who were treated for at least 3 days recovered, and with recovery their IFN responses returned to normal. In the late 1960s it was reported that no IFN could be found in the blood of 'infectious' or 'serum' hepatitis patients[41]. Some subsequent studies have confirmed these observations, but at the same time there is evidence that circulating IFN may be present in some cases in the acute stage[42]. We evaluated 73 cases of acute hepatitis and found a mean (±SE) blood IFN of 43±7 units/ml compared to 76±10 units/ml in patients with other viral illnesses. The main difference between the two groups was that a higher percentage of hepatitis patients had zero blood IFN levels (30%) than those with other viral infections (<5%), and the same held true for *in vitro* IFN-α and IFN-γ production[43]. In fulminant hepatitis, 56% had no detectable IFN in the blood.

In a report 10 years ago it was found that children with chronic HB hepatitis had reduced *in vitro* IFN-α production[44], and subsequently others have confirmed these findings[45]. However, we found that most of the chronic hepatitis patients whom we studied had normal IFN responses, and very few had low responses.

In summary, it appears that some patients who become infected with hepatitis viruses are unable to generate a normal IFN response during the acute stage of the illness. This is a temporary phenomenon. In rare cases the deficiency may be complete, encompassing both *in vivo* and *in vitro* IFN responses, and these cases usually have a progressive disease with a fatal outcome.

Defective IFN production by PBMC has been reported in patients with pre-leukaemia, acute non-lymphocytic leukaemia with acquired abnormalities of chromosome 5[46] and in chronic lymphatic leukaemia[30, 47]. In hairy-cell leukaemia (HCL), IFN-α production alone was found to be very low on repeated assays, and it is suggested that this is due to diminution of monocytes which are a main source of IFN-α production[48]. A suggestion that HCL is an IFN deficient disease was made by a group of workers in Switzerland based on evidence that rIFN-α is an effective therapy in this condition; in almost every case the cytopenia was reversed although complete eradication of hairy cells from the bone marrow was rarely obtained[49]. This therapeutic effect can then be maintained by relatively small doses of IFN given once a week.

Patients with systemic lupus erythematosus, particularly during the active stage, have defective *in vitro* IFN-α but normal IFN-γ production in response to a number of viral stimulants[50]. In patients with multiple sclerosis (MS), a different type of IFN deficiency has been reported, namely the ineffectiveness of these patients' *in vitro* IFN-α response to specific viral and other antigens such as measles virus, NDV and Poly-IC[51]. Later it was shown that MS patients under treatment with IFN-α produced somewhat less IFN-α than prior to therapy when their PBMC were stimulated with these agents[52]. However, our own study of 30 MS patients in various stages of disease activity showed that most tended to have activated IFN systems with normal *in vitro* IFN-α and IFN-γ production, a pattern seen in patients with viral illnesses[53].

THERAPEUTIC USE OF INTERFERON

From the beginning of the IFN era the IFN produced for therapeutic purposes was prepared from virus-stimulated human leukocytes according to a method first described by Cantell[54]. The supernatant fluid was collected, concentrated, purified and sterilized and originally gave a final product of IFN which was only about 1% pure. There is no doubt that lymphokines, other than a mixture of IFN-α classes, were present in this material. We, for example, have detected significant amounts of leukotriene C4 and traces of IL-2 in our IFN-α preparation. About 3–10 million units can be obtained from the stimulated buffy-coat of a single blood unit. When ready for use, it is usually supplied in sterile vials containing 3 mega units/ml (2–5 mega units/mg protein) for intramuscular or intravenous use. The HuIFN-α used in our studies was produced and supplied to us by The Israel Biological Research Institute in Nes Ziona. IFN-α is also produced following stimulation of lymphoblasts (Namalva line) by virus, with further purification required to remove all traces of DNA of the producing cell. IFN-β is similarly produced from supernatants of fibroblasts induced by virus. It appears that T lymphocytes, and more specifically T4-helper cells are the primary, but not only source of IFN-γ. This class of IFN is much more difficult to produce, and supplies of the natural substance have always been limited. In this instance viruses are not used as inducers, rather proteinaceous stimulants such as PHA, *Staph. enterotoxin A* and Con-A.

The problems of limited supplies of interferons and their high costs were overcome in 1980 with the successful adaptation of recombinant DNA technology for IFN production. Today numerous IFNs of the α, β and γ classes are being produced by clones of bacteria programmed to produce human IFN in large quantities in commercial laboratories; hopefully this will lead to a fall in the price. At the time of preparing this review, rIFN-αA is the preparation in most common use, particularly in cancer patients where large amounts are required for extended courses of treatment.

In the doses usually recommended for the treatment of acute viral diseases (3 mega units/day or 70 000 units $kg^{-1} day^{-1}$ for babies) side-effects are minimal and usually only consist of transient fever 2–4 hours after the first few injections. Occasionally symptoms suggestive of mild influenzae have been reported, but treatment can nevertheless be continued. At this dosage, granulocytopenia and thrombocytopenia are rarely seen and are anyway reversible by stopping the treatment.

SUMMARY

It appears that defective IFN production by cells can occur in numerous diseases and conditions, often secondary to changes in the blood mononuclear cells. This is often transient and usually involves only a part of the IFN production system. On recovery, the IFN system returns to normal. The clinical significance of this transient and partial defect is not clear. However, when both IFN-α and IFN-γ production by PBMC are totally defective and no IFN is produced *in vivo* in the course of an acute viral infection, then an antiviral state of cells does not develop and the viral disease progresses and usually ends in death. If the deficiency is recognized and IFN therapy begun, the disease can be brought under control with complete clinical recovery, unless irreversible tissue or organ damage has already occurred. It seems that this deficiency state is more common with certain viruses, such as hepatitis viruses, herpes infections and possibly measles. In suspected cases of unremittent progressive viral disease, it is logical to give IFN-α as early as possible, even if a specific laboratory diagnosis is not available.

References

1. Isaacs, A. and Lindenmann, J. (1957). Virus interference. 1. The interferon. 2. Some properties of interferon. *Proc. R. Soc. Lond. (Biol).*, **147**, 258-73
2. Henle, W. and Henle, G. (1984). The road to interferon interference by inactivated influenza virus. In Billiou, A. (ed.) *Interferon: General and Applied Aspects*. pp. 3-22. (Amsterdam: Elsevier Press)
3. Stewart, W. E. II. (1979). *The Interferon System*. (New York: Springer-Verlag)
4. Levin, S. and Hahn, T. (1981). Evaluation of the interferon system in viral disease. *Clin. Exp. Immunol.*, **46**, 475-83
5. Grossberg, S. E. and Taylor, G. L. (1984). Interferon effects on cell differentiation. In Friedman, R. M. (ed.) *Interferon. 3. Mechanism of Production and Action*. pp. 299-317. (Amsterdam: Elsevier)
6. Vilcek, J. and De Maeyer, F. (1984). *Interferon. 2. Interferons and the Immune System*. (Amsterdam: Elsevier)
7. Stiehm, E. R. and Fulginiti, V. A. (1980). *Immunological Disorders in Infants and Children*. 2nd edn. (Philadelphia: W. B. Saunders)
8. Levin, S. and Hahn, T. (1985). Interferon deficiency syndrome. *Clin. Exp. Immunol.*, **60**, 267-73
9. Levin, S., Hahn, T. and Handzel, Z. T. (1985). Activated interferon system in healthy homosexual men. *Antiviral Res.*, **5**, 229-40
10. Mims, C. A. (1986). Interactions of viruses with the immune system. *Clin. Exp. Immunol.*, **66**, 1-16
11. Saksela, E. (1981). Interferon and natural killer cells. In Gresser, I. (ed.) *Interferon*. Vol 3. pp. 45-63. (London: Academic Press)
12. Breese Hall, C., Douglas, R. G., Simons, R. L. and Geiman, J. M. (1978). Interferon production in children with respiratory syncytial, influenza and parainfluenza infections. *J. Pediatr.*, **93**, 28-32
13. Hahn, T. and Levin, S. (1982). The interferon system in patients with malignant disease. *J. Interferon Res.*, **2**, 97-102
14. Levin, S. and Hahn, T. (1980). The interferon system in immunodeficiency and deficiency of the interferon system. In Seligman, M. and Hitzig, W. H. (eds.) *Primary Immunodeficiencies*. pp. 465-72. (Amsterdam: Elsevier/North Holland)
15. Isaacs, D., Tyrrel, D. A. S., Clarke, J. R., Webster, A. D. B. and Valman, H. B. (1981). Deficient production of leucocyte interferon *in vitro* and *in vivo* in children with recurrent respiratory tract infections. *Lancet*, **2**, 950-2
16. Murray, H. W., Rubin, B. Y., Masur, H. and Roberts, R. B. (1984). Impaired production of lymphokines and immune (gamma) interferon in AIDS. *N. Engl. J. Med.*, **310**, 883-9
17. Virelizier, J. L. and Griscelli, C. (1981). Selective defect of interferon secretion associated with impaired natural killing activity. *Arch. Fr. Pediat.*, **38**, 77-81
18. Virelizier, J. L., Lenoir, G. and Griscelli, C. (1978). Persistent EBV infection in a child with

hypergammaglobulinaemia and immunoblastic proliferation associated with a selective defect in immune interferon secretion. *Lancet*, **2**, 231-4

19. Virelizier, J. L., Lipinski, M., Tursz, T. and Griscelli, C. (1979). Defects of immune interferon secretion and natural killer activity in patients with immunological disorders. *Lancet*, **2**, 696-7
20. Stiehm, E. R. (Moderator) (1982). Interferon: immunobiology and clinical significance. UCLA conference. *Ann. Intern. Med.*, **96**, 80-93
21. Hahn, T., Levin, S. and Handzel, Z. T. (1980). Production of immune and viral interferon by lymphocytes of newborn infants. *Isr. J. Med. Sci.*, **16**, 33-6
22. Bryson, Y. J., Winter, H. S., Gard, S. E., Fischer, T. J. and Stiehm, E. R. (1980). Deficiency of immune interferon production by leucocytes of normal newborns. *Cell Immunol.*, **55**, 191-200
23. Wakasugi, N., Virelizier, J. L. *et al.* (1985). Defective IFN-γ production in the human neonate. *J. Immunol.*, **134**, 167-76
24. Rytel, M. W., Larratt, K. S., Turner, P. A. and Kalbfleisch, J. H. (1986). Interferon response to mitogens and viral antigens in elderly and young adult subjects. *J. Infect. Dis.*, **153**, 984-7
25. Epstein, L. B. and Ammann, A. J. (1974). Evaluation of T lymphocyte effector function in immunodeficiency disease: abnormality in mitogen-stimulated interferon in patients with selective IgA deficiency. *J. Immunol.*, **112**, 617-26
26. Miller, M. E. and Hummeler, K. (1967). Thymic dysplasia (Swiss agammaglobulinemia). 2. Morphologic and functional observations. *J. Pediatr.*, **70**, 737
27. Ray, C. G. and Starkey, D. D. (1970). Leucocyte interferon production in immunological deficiency diseases. *Lancet*, **1**, 312
28. Aiuti, F., Capobianchi, M. R., Dianzani, F. *et al.* (1983). Interferon gamma production in patients with primary immunodeficiency. In *The Interferon System. Program and abstracts*, Rome, p. 132
29. Levin, S., Schlesinger, M., Handzel, Z. T. and Hahn, T. (1979). Thymic deficiency in Down's syndrome. *Pediatrics*, **63**, 80-7
30. Strander, J., Cantell, K., Leisti, J. and Nikkila, E. (1970). Interferon response of lymphocytes in disorders with decreased resistance to infections. *Clin. Exp. Immunol.*, **6**, 263-72
31. Guillou, P. J., Giles, G. R. and Ramsden, C. W. (1986). Natural killer-cell activity, interferon-α2 production, and interleukin-2 production in cyclosporine-treated and conventionally immunosuppressed human allograft recipients. *J. Clin. Immunol.*, **6**, 373-80
32. Bacon, T. H., de Vere-Tyndall, A., Tyrrell, D. A. J. *et al.* (1983). Interferon system in patients with systemic juvenile chronic arthritis: *in vivo* and *in vitro* studies. *Clin. Exp. Immunol.*, **54**, 23-30
33. Adolph, G. R. and Swetley, P. (1979). Glucocorticoid hormones inhibit DNA synthesis and enhance interferon production in a human lymphoid cell line. *Nature (London)*, **282**, 736
34. Emodi, G. and Just, M. (1974). Impaired interferon response of children with congenital cytomegalovirus disease. *Acta Paediatr. Scand.*, **63**, 183-7
35. Rozee, K. R., Lee, S. H. S. *et al.* (1982). Is a compromised interferon response an etiologic factor in Reye's syndrome? *Can. Med. Assoc. J.*, **126**, 798-802
36. Klieman, R. L., Green, J. A. and Spruance, S. L. (1985). Immunostimulatory function of herpes simplex isolates from patients with frequent herpes labialis and a deficiency in immune specific interferon production. *J. Med. Virol.*, **16**, 289-96
37. Bondestam, M., Funa, K. and Alm, G. F. (1985). Defective leukocyte interferon response in children with recurrent infections accompanied by arthralgia. *Acta Paediatr. Scand.*, **74**, 219-25
38. Viljek, J., Klion, A. *et al.* (1986). Defective gamma-interferon production in peripheral blood leukocytes of patients with acute tuberculosis. *J. Clin. Immunol.*, **6**, 146-51
39. Huygen, K., Mascort-Lemore, F., Cran, S. *et al.* (1985). Analysis of the interferon system in African patients with acquired immunodeficiency syndrome. *Eur. J. Clin Microbiol.*, **4**, 304-9
40. Hersch, E. M., Gutterman, J. U., Spector, S. *et al.* (1985). Impaired *in vitro* interferon, blastogenic and natural killer cell responses to viral stimulation in AIDS. *Cancer Res.*, **45**, 406-10
41. Levin, S. and Hahn, T. (1982). Interferon system in acute viral hepatitis. *Lancet*, 592-4

42. Bador, H., Colobert, L., Giroud, M. and Lesbre, F. (1977). Production d'interferon et participation de l'a2-macroglobuline a la response immunologique au cours de l'hepatite humane de type A. *Clin. Chem. Acta*, **78**, 217-26
43. Levin, S. (1987). Interferon-alpha treatment in acute progressive and fulminant hepatitis. Presented at the *International Symposium on the Immunology of the Gastrointestinal Tract and the Liver*, March 22-27, Jerusalem
44. Tolentino, P., Dianzani, F., Zucca, M. and Giacchino, R. (1975). Decreased interferon response by lymphocytes from children with chronic hepatitis. *J. Infect. Dis.*, **132**, 459-61
45. Ikeda, T., Pignatelli, M., Thomas, H. C. *et al.* (1985). An alpha-interferon deficiency state exists in some patients with chronic hepatitis B infection. *Hepatology*, **5**, 988
46. Pedersen-Bjergaard, J., Haahr, S., Philip, P., Thomsen, M., Jensen, G., Ersboll, J. and Nissen, N. I. (1980). Abolished production of interferon by lymphocytes of patients with the acquired cytogenic abnormalities 5q-or-5p in secondary and *de novo* acute non-lymphocytic leukemia. *Br. J. Haemat.*, **46**, 211-33
47. Ludwig, H. (1979). Absent serum interferon in chronic lymphatic leukemia. *N. Engl. J. Med.*, **301**, 1007
48. Porzolt, F., Janik, R., Heil, G. *et al.* (1986). Deficient interferon-alpha production in hairy-cell leukemia. *Blut*, **52**, 185-90
49. Hofmann, V., Fehr, J., Sauter, C. and Ottino, J. (1985). Hairy cell leukemia, an interferon deficient disease? *Cancer Treatment Rev.*, **12**, 33-7
50. Neighbour, P. A. and Grayzel, A. L. (1981). Interferon production *in vitro* by leucocytes from patients with systemic lupus erythematosus and rheumatoid arthritis. *Clin. Exp. Immunol.*, **45**, 576-82
51. Neighbour, P. A. and Bloom B. R. (1979). Absence of virus-induced lymphocyte suppression and interferon production in multiple sclerosis. *Proc. Natl. Acad. Sci. USA.*, **76**, 476-80
52. Kamin-Lewis, R. M., Panitch, H. S., Merigan, T. C. and Johnson, K. P. (1984). Decreased interferon synthesis and responsiveness to interferon by leukocytes from multiple sclerosis patients given natural alpha interferon. *J. Interferon Res.*, **3**, 423-32
53. Kott, E., Levin, S., Huberman, M. and Hahn, T. (1982). Human leucocyte interferon in patients with multiple sclerosis: interferon system and NK activity in multiple sclerosis. *Neurology*, **32**, 47
54. Kauppinen, H. L. (1985). Sources of interferon for clinical use: α-interferons from blood leucocytes. In Finter, N. B. and Oldhan, R. K. (eds.) *Interferon. 4. In vivo and clinical studies.* pp. 73-9. (Amsterdam: Elsevier)

8
Neutrophil and Complement Defects: Recent Advances

A. SEGAL AND M. WALPORT

INTRODUCTION

Although a great deal has been learnt about the physiology of phagocytic cells and the complement system from *in vitro* studies, one cannot necessarily relate such findings to their physiological importance *in vivo*. It is only by the study of patients with well defined abnormalities of complement or phagocyte function that one can learn how these systems actually function *in vivo*. Of particular value have been the studies of patients with inherited deficiencies of single proteins. Patients with neutrophil and monocyte abnormalities frequently suffer from recurrent pyogenic infections, those with complement deficiencies develop recurrent infections and also have a high prevalence of immune complex disease. Although patients with inherited deficiencies are extremely rare, nevertheless they have taught us a great deal about the normal biology of both phagocytic cells and the complement system. Such patients represent 'experiments of nature' and the frequency with which such individuals are encountered is often inversely related to the impact they have upon our understanding of the biology of phagocytic cells, the complement system and their role in host defence.

PHAGOCYTE DYSFUNCTION

Phagocytic cells play the primary role in protecting the body against infection by bacteria, fungi and parasites. They also remove and digest exogenous and endogenous debris in the tissues. The most obvious manifestation of the impaired function of these cells is an unusual predisposition to infection. Because ostensibly normal individuals are also susceptible to infection, it is usually only after unusually frequent or inappropriately severe or protracted infections, or invasion by an unusual organism, in an individual or family, that a deficiency of host defence is considered.

These infections most commonly involve anatomical areas particularly exposed to bacterial colonization, including the skin, upper respiratory tract and lungs, mouth and gums, and perineum. Infection is also common in the liver, lymph nodes and bone marrow. Presumably in these situations the microbes are initially cleared from the circulation by cells of the reticuloendothelial system in which they multiply having failed to be killed.

A great many conditions, including pregnancy, the neonatal period, thermal injury, malnutrition and malignancy, have been reported in association with phagocytic cell dysfunction[1,2]. In these circumstances the aetiology of the lesion is variable and multifactorial, making it almost impossible to define the precise mechanism involved. In contrast, in inherited defects the abnormal mechanism can generally be attributed to a single abnormal protein, the functional significance of which can then be more clearly understood. In this chapter we will concentrate on a few well defined inherited lesions that have taught us a great deal about the normal biology of these cells.

CHRONIC GRANULOMATOUS DISEASE

Introduction

Enormous strides have recently been made in the elucidation of the molecular processes involved in the pathogenesis of chronic granulomatous disease (CGD). An entire volume has been recently devoted to this condition[3].

Clinical manifestations

The patients with this syndrome are unduly susceptible to infection[4] because of impaired killing of certain organisms by their phagocytes[5]. Phagocytosis by these cells seems to clear the blood and tissues of organisms, which remain viable when they are taken up by the reticuloendothelial system. The inital presentation is often with adenitis, usually in the inguinal glands in infants when nappies (diapers) are worn and then in the cervical region. Liver abscess and osteomyelitis are also relatively common in these patients. The respiratory tract and skin are also frequent sites of infection. Drainage or discharge from an infected site is often associated with delayed healing, sinus formation and scarring. This clinical presentation coupled with the histological picture of granulomata often results in a mistaken diagnosis of mycobacterial infection.

Staphylococci are the commonest infecting organisms, but some very unusual microbes like *Serratia marcescens* and fungi may be responsible[6].

Although the molecular defect is congenital and constant the frequency and severity of infection varies considerably from patient to patient. It is not uncommon for these patients to first present with major infection in the second decade or later.

The microbicidal oxidase system of phagocytic cells

This system is the site of the primary abnormality in CGD. In order to appreciate the molecular basis of CGD it is necessary to understand the nature and function of this system.

The professional phagocytic cells, neutrophils, monocytes, macrophages and eosinophils, demonstrate a very unusual process when they engulf microbes. They rapidly consume relatively large amounts of oxygen[7,8] which is not used to generate energy by mitochondrial oxidative phosphorylation for phagocytosis. Phagocytosis occurs quite normally in the absence of oxygen, and this respiratory burst is not inhibited by mitochondrial poisons such as cyanide or azide[9].

This unusual oxygen consumption is required to produce the optimal conditions for the killing of most common bacterial and fungal pathogens as well as a variety of commensals. The importance of this respiration in microbicidal processes is demonstrated by a reduced efficiency of killing of certain microbes by normal cells deprived of oxygen[10,11], and by the syndrome of CGD in which the phagocytes of these patients show a similar inability to kill the same organisms coupled with a complete absence of this respiratory activity[12].

The oxidase system

The overall reaction transfers electrons from the high energy state of glucose to oxygen. The electrons from glucose are first incorporated into the low potential, high energy, reduced pyridine nucleotide, NADPH[13]. These electrons are then transferred to high potential, low energy oxygen by means of an electron transport chain[14].

The only well characterized component of this chain is a very unusual cytochrome b, called b-245 because of its mid-point potential of -245 mV[15]. It has also been labelled b_{558}, which refers to the wavelength of the α peak of absorbance, but this is less discriminating because a number of other cytochromes b also absorb maximally at this wavelength. This cytochrome is located in the membrane of the specific granules of neutrophils and in the plasma membrane of these cells and the other phagocytes[16,17], and is incorporated into the wall of the phagocytic vacuole as this forms[18]. It is probably the terminal component of this electron transport chain. It binds CO, a strong indication that it can bind oxygen[19], transfers electrons from NADPH to this oxygen at precisely the rate of superoxide generation[20] and its unusually low mid-point potential provides it with the bioenergetic capability to pass electrons directly to oxygen to form superoxide. Another unusual feature is that it has two protein subunits[21] with molecular weights of 76–92 kDa and 23 kDa. The larger subunit is heavily glycosylated[22], suggesting an external location on the plasma membrane. The multiple subunits and CO binding are atypical features of mammalian cytochromes, but are features of bacterial cytochromes[23].

There must be other components in the chain because cytochromes are unable to receive electrons directly from NADPH. There is some evidence for the presence of a flavoprotein containing FAD as cofactor, but it has proved difficult to identify the specific molecule, probably because there are a number of different flavoproteins in these cells and their measurement is less

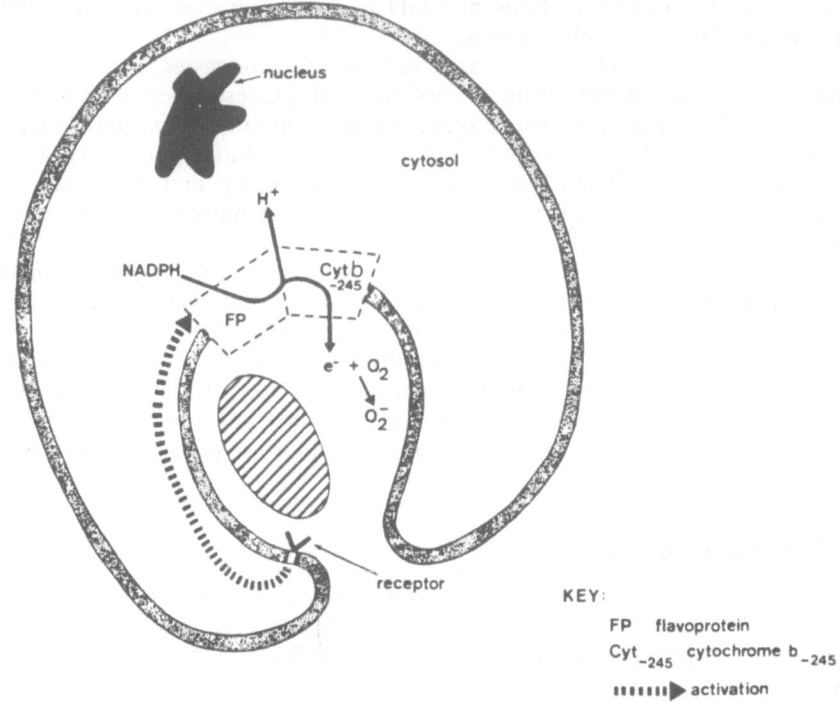

Figure 8.1 Schematic representation of microbicidal oxidase of phagocytes. This is an electron transport chain composed of a flavoprotein dehydrogenase and cytochrome b-245 that is situated in the wall of the phagocytic vacuole. It takes electrons from the substrate NADPH and transfers them to oxygen to generate superoxide in the vacuole. The superoxide dismutates to form peroxide which disproportionates to the protonated state, consuming protons and elevating the vacuolar pH

precise than that of cytochromes. Some preparations of the solubilized oxidase have been shown to contain FAD[24] whereas oxidase activity is abrogated by the competitive inhibitor, 5-deazaFAD[25].

Some investigators have identified ubiquinone in extracts of neutrophils[26–28], but this is probably derived from the mitochondria of contaminating platelets and mononuclear cells[29].

Hence, the path of electrons in this microbicidal oxidase is probably from glucose to NADPH via the hexose monophosphate shunt, and then from a flavoprotein to cytochrome b-245 and finally onto oxygen (Figure 8.1).

The molecular basis of CGD

The phenotypic hallmark of the CGD syndrome is complete absence of this oxidase system. This unifying mechanism can result from a wide range of genetically distinct molecular lesions[30]. There are two main patterns of inheritance, the commoner X-linked, and autosomal recessive. The existence of very different causal mechanisms is beautifully demonstrated by the correction of the molecular lesions when cells from patients with different patterns of inheritance are fused together[31].

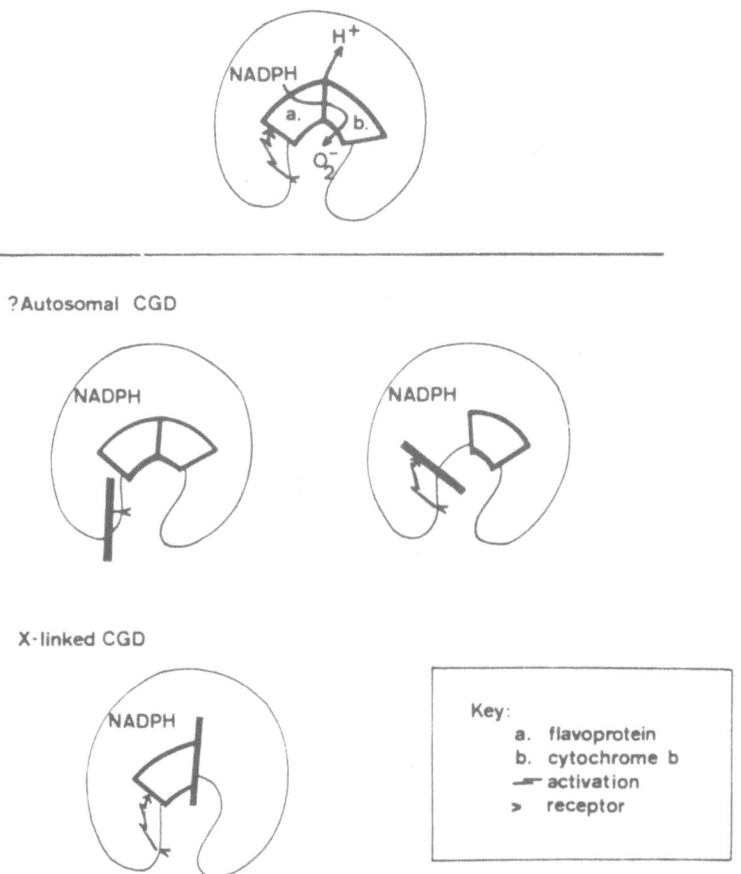

Figure 8.2 The relationship between cytochrome b-245 and the different subtypes of chronic granulomatous disease. (Above) Activation with phorbol myristate acetate (PMA) switches on the oxidase by causing the alternate oxidation and reduction of the redox components of the chain. When oxygen is eliminated from the system the electrons are not removed, and the components of the chain become arrested in the reduced state. (Below) When converted from the oxidized to the reduced state, cytochrome b-245 undergoes a characteristic change in colour that can be measured with a spectrophotometer. This reduction can be accomplished chemically, for example with dithionite, or by activating the cells in the absence of oxygen. In normal cells both forms of reduction reduce the cytochrome and produce the characteristic spectrum. After chemical reduction the cytochrome is undetectable in X-linked CGD, indicating that this is the site of the lesion. In subjects with an autosomal pattern of inheritance chemical reduction reveals the cytochrome, but failure of autoreduction indicates defective activation of the electron transport chain or the absence of one of its components proximal to the cytochrome

Inheritance on the X chromosome

The largest subgroup of patients inherit an X-linked defect, with affected males and heterozygote carrier females. The molecular basis of the lesion in the vast majority of these patients is the absence of cytochrome b-245 from their phagocytes[32, 33] (Figure 8.2), which are missing the haem spectrum and both the α and β polypeptide chains of this molecule[21]. The heterozygote carriers have intermediate amounts of the cytochrome and a close relationship exists between the depressed level and the proportion of cells in which the normal X-chromosome is suppressed by Lyonization.

A freak patient has been described in whom a deletion of a short segment of the short arm of the X chromosome resulted in the combined abnormalities of Duchenne muscular dystrophy, retinitis pigmentosa and CGD (with absence of detectable neutrophil cytochrome b)[34]; it is probable that the abnormality in most of these X-linked subjects is a point mutation in this region of the chromosome. A gene has been cloned which appears to be abnormal in these patients[35]. Although the protein for which it codes has yet to be identified it does not appear to be the apoprotein of either subunit of the cytochrome. It could be some other component of the electron transport chain or a related structural or controlling protein.

Autosomal recessive inheritance

The molecular defect is very different in these subjects. Although their cells contain normal amounts of the cytochrome, and its properties and subcellular distribution appear normal, they are unable to transfer electrons onto it[32, 36] (Figure 8.3). This could be explained by an abnormality of the activation processes or the absence or abnormality of a proximal link in the electron transport chain (Figure 8.2).

Activation mechanisms in neutrophils are currently the focus of intense interest[37]. One of the major common pathways seems to be through the phosphorylation of the target protein by protein kinase C[38], which is directly activated by phorbol myristate acetate, a potent stimulator of the oxidase system.

Recent studies have shown that this process is defective in most of these subjects. Their cells demonstrate a consistent failure to phosphorylate a protein band with an apparent molecular weight of 47 kDa[39]. It is probable that this phosphoprotein is involved in the oxidase system, possibly even the proximal flavoprotein dehydrogenase itself. The failure to phosphorylate it could reflect an absence of the protein, a point mutation leading to loss of the amino acid target of phosphorylation, usually serine or threonine, or malfunction of a specific protein kinase.

Others

Lack of NADPH, the substrate of this oxidase system, can lead to a CGD-like state. This occurs as a result of a very severe deficiency of G-6-P-D, a key enzyme in the hexose monophosphate shunt responsible for generating NADPH[40].

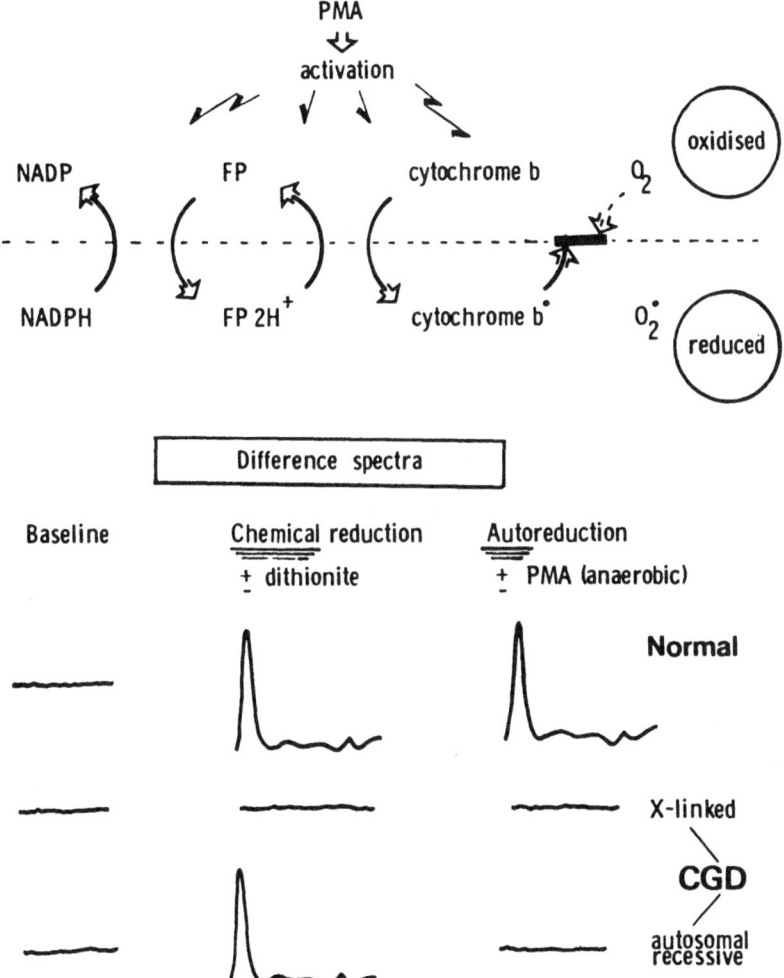

Figure 8.3 Schematic representation of the probable structure of the electron transport chain (above) and site of the lesion in CGD with the autosomal recessive and X-linked patterns of inheritance (below)

A very unusual patient has been described whose cells failed to show the respiratory burst during phagocytosis, whereas normal oxidase activity was elicited by stimulation with PMA, indicating a lesion between the receptor and activation of protein kinase C[41]. It is probable that a number of other isolated lesions causing CGD, each with their own story to tell, will be discovered.

The basis of the microbicidal defect in CGD

The respiratory burst is essential for the effective killing of certain common pathogenic bacteria and fungi. Under anaerobic conditions[10, 11], and in CGD[5], these organisms are phagocytosed normally but a percentage of them remain viable within the phagocytic vacuole[5, 42].

There are three main mechanisms by which this respiration might promote killing (Figure 8.4) and they almost certainly interact synergistically.

Free radical generation

The donation by cytochrome b-245 of a single electron to oxygen results in the formation of superoxide[43], which dismutates to form hydrogen peroxide[44]. The discovery of this phenomenon led to speculation that these reduced oxygen species may themselves be toxic to the organisms. However, the development of cytoplasts[45], preparations of neutrophils from which the granules and nuclei have been removed, has allowed this to be studied by providing a model for separating the radical generating system from the granule contents. These bodies phagocytose and demonstrate a normal respiratory burst but bacterial killing is impaired[45] (E. Odell, unpublished) indicating a requirement for the granule contents in the killing process. It is possible, but unlikely, that they do this through the potentiation of radical damage. Iron is a potent catalyst for the generation of hydroxyl radicals. Opinion differs as to whether lactoferrin potentiates[46] the generation of these radicals by supplying iron, or inhibits it by chelation[47].

Myeloperoxidase-mediated halogenation

Neutrophils contain a relatively large amount of myeloperoxidase (MPO), accounting for about 5% of the total protein of the cell. Its function has not been clearly elucidated. It has the potential to use hydrogen peroxide as substrate to oxidize halides like chloride and iodide to chlorine and iodine and their hypohalous acids[48], but whether this is a major physiological pathway is unclear. MPO reacts with O_2^- in the phagocytic vacuole and has the ability to degrade H_2O_2 to H_2O through a catalase-like mechanism, and may only halogenate at low concentrations of peroxide[49]. It is certainly not essential for immunity because large numbers of symptomless subjects have been identified whose cells are completely devoid of this enzyme.

Alkalinization of the phagocytic vacuole

The neutrophil granules contain proteins, particularly a group which are strongly cationic, that are potently microbicidal *in vitro*[50]. The puzzle is that the same proteins are much less effective when released onto the organism within the environment of the phagocytic vacuole in the cell of a patient with CGD. This must indicate a difference within this environment. Most of the early work on lysosomes was conducted on liver cells in which the operative pH in these organelles is very low[51]. Largely by analogy, it has been accepted that it should also be acid in the phagocytic vacuoles of phagocytes. Early

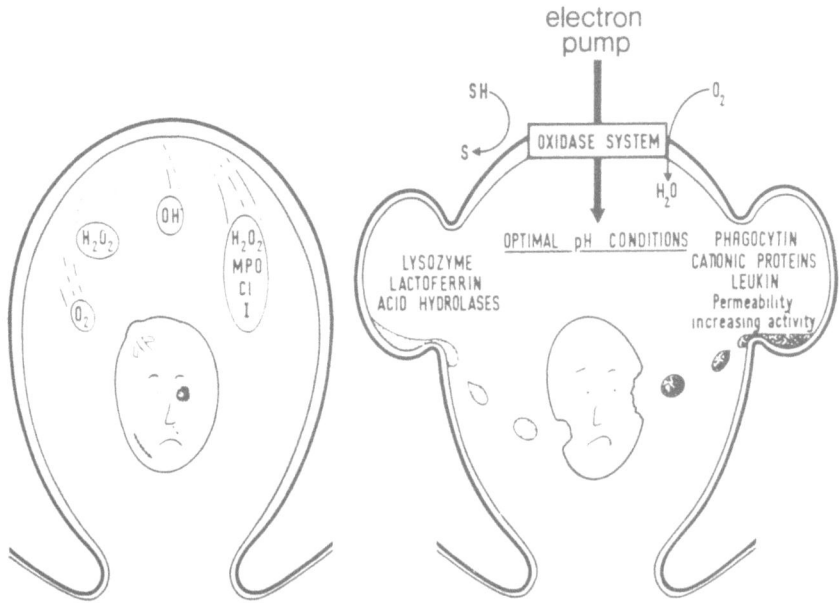

Figure 8.4 Possible mechanisms by which the oxidase may contribute to bacterial killing in the phagocytic vacuole. The oxidase generates a variety of species of reduced oxygen which could be directly toxic or provide the substrate for myeloperoxidase-mediated halogenation. Alternatively, the oxidase could elevate the pH within the phagocytic vacuole to that optimal for the effective antimicrobial activity of the granule proteins. These three processes probably operate synergistically

studies with pH sensitive dyes coupled to phagocytosed particles confirmed this acidity[52], but they were only detecting relatively late events.

In fact the pH within this compartment in normal cells undergoes a remarkable initial rise to about 7.8–8.0 before gradually drifting down to about 6.0[42, 53, 54]. The probable reason for this elevation is that the electron transport chain is pumping electrons, unaccompanied by protons, into the vacuole. The reduced oxygen products, superoxide and peroxide, are both anionic and consume protons as they disproportionate to the protonated form.

In CGD, and in the absence of oxygen, this early elevation of pH is not observed and the pH falls precipitously to about 1.5 pH units lower than normal[42]. This is important because it has been demonstrated that bacterial killing by the granule cationic proteins only occurs at pHs above 7.0[50]. This would explain why CGD cells kill most, but not all, ingested organisms[55]. Microbes entering the vacuole early after phagocytosis will be exposed to granule contents while the pH is still relatively neutral and will be killed, whereas those that are slightly more resistant or are sequestered within a clump of organisms, might survive until the pH has fallen to less optimal levels.

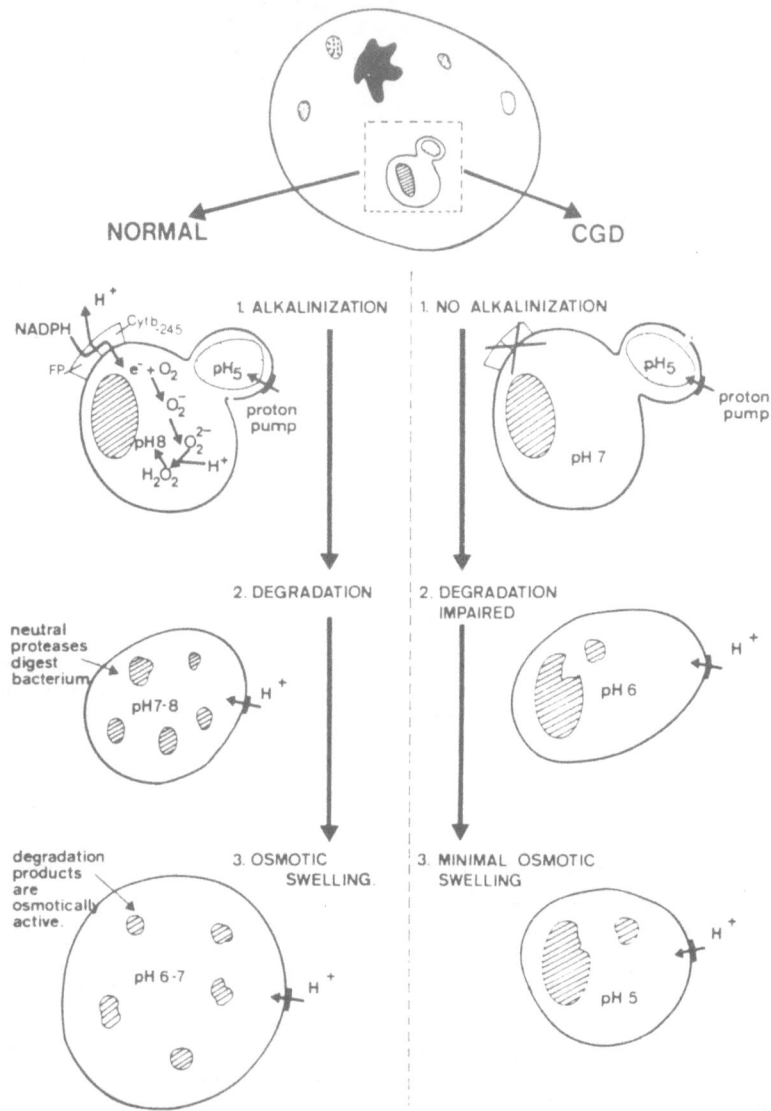

Figure 8.5 Probable sequence of events controlling pH within the phagocytic vacuole. Initially the pH will be the same as that of the extracellular medium engulfed together with the particle. The electron transport chain then pumps electrons attached to oxygen into the vacuole in the form of superoxide. The superoxide, and the product of its dismutation, peroxide, become protonated, and this consumption of protons elevates the vacuolar pH. The granule proteins, which are maintained inactive at low pH, probably by a proton pump like that in the wall of the chromaffin granule[64], are suddenly activated by this alkaline environment. They kill and digest the microbes and the osmotically active products of digestion attract water into the vacuole which swells. In CGD the granules fuse with the vacuole, releasing their acid contents into the lumen, the pH of which consequently falls. This low pH inhibits the granule enzymes, impairing killing and digestion, with an absence of the associated osmotic swelling

Digestion

Neutrophil, monocyte and macrophage granules contain a potent array of digestive enzymes that are largely active at neutral pH[56], and are important for the degradation of microbial and autologous debris. The abnormal acidity of the phagocytic vacuoles in CGD impairs this function[42] (Figure 8.5), resulting in the accumulation of indigestable debris. The granulomata that are the hallmark of this condition are not in the main a reflection of persistent infection, but rather an indication of a normal response to the accumulation of undegradable material. Some of these subjects develop a massive hepatosplenomegaly, while these organs are not palpably enlarged in others. The reason for this variability is unclear. These organs contain lipid-filled histiocytes[57], and the original description of the histology in CGD concluded that the appearances more closely resembled a storage disease, like Niemann–Pick disease, than infection, but were unable to explain the mechanism by which this might occur[57]. We can now see that it is in fact a storage disease resulting from a failure of the degradative enzymes. However, in this instance it is not due to an absence of the hydrolytic enzyme, but because it fails to function efficiently in a suboptimal environment.

Diagnosis

The diagnosis is very simple once it has been considered. It depends upon the demonstration of the complete absence of oxidase activity from the patient's phagocytes. This can be accomplished by a variety of techniques, but the simplest screening methods are probably the NBT slide[58] or column[59] tests, and chemiluminescence[60]. In either event it is important that the diagnosis is verified in a different system, such as superoxide-dependent cytochrome c reduction[61], and that care is taken to ensure that the cells have been given a supra-maximal stimulus (e.g. $1 \mu g / ml$ PMA) that exerts its action beyond the receptor stage.

It is then useful to establish the molecular basis of the condition and mode of inheritance. An X-linked inheritance in a male is demonstrated by the observation of a mosaic of normal and abnormal cells in the circulation of the mother and a proportion of the female relatives in the maternal family. This mosaicism is best identified by the NBT slide test[58].

The presence or absence of cytochrome b-245 is determined by difference spectroscopy[62] of purified neutrophils.

The NBT slide test can also be used on umbilical cord blood for the antenatal diagnosis of CGD.

Molecular biological techniques should soon provide major advances in our understanding of the genotypic basis and inheritance of this condition, as well as improved and earlier antenatal diagnosis.

Treatment

The current basis of treatment is continuous prophylaxis with co-trimoxazole in standard therapeutic doses. Hypersensitivity reactions occur quite commonly, in which circumstance the sulphamethoxazole is omitted and prophylaxis maintained with trimethoprim alone.

Active infections must be treated promptly and aggressively. Particular effort must be made to identify the offending organism. This poses a special problem in the case of patchy pneumonia where failure to grow the organism from sputum should be followed by bronchoscopy with bronchial washing and transbronchial biopsy, and if this proves negative, with open lung biopsy.

Intercurrent infections are treated with the appropriate chemotherapy, and where available with infusions of normal neutrophils obtained by leuko-phoresis or from buffy-coat residues.

It might be possible to correct the abnormally acidic conditions within the phagocytic vacuoles of these patients, and thereby reverse the defective killing and digestion, with drugs such as amantidine, weak bases and chloroquine.

In the long term CGD should be amenable to gene therapy.

CHEDIAK-HIGASHI DISEASE

This syndrome is characterized by frequent pyogenic infection, partial oculocutaneous albinism and a peripheral neuropathy. It progresses to an 'accclerated' lymphoma-like phase with hepatosplenomegaly, widespread lymphoid and histiocytic infiltrates, and pancytopenia, which is usually terminal.

The neutrophils appear to be continuously activated, respiring and phagocytosing in the unstimulated state. The diagnostic feature is the presence of giant cytoplasmic ganules in the leukocytes. These giant inclusions do not appear to be a developmental anomaly, but rather a result of the fusion of the granules to form enormous secondary lysosomes[63]. This results in a relative deficiency of the microbicidal granule contents available for release into new phagocytic vacuoles containing engulfed microbes.

Bone marrow transplantation offers the only feasible treatment for this condition.

COMPLEMENT DEFICIENCY AND DISEASE

Inherited deficiences of the majority of the components of the complement system are now well described and have recently been extensively reviewed[65-67]. Here we will concentrate on presenting recent findings on the mechanisms of complement deficiency and attempt to explain some of the disease associations. Deficiencies, both inherited and acquired, of complement receptors have recently been described and these are considered in detail below.

Disease associations

Classical pathway components

Inherited complete deficiencies of C1q, C1r, C1s, C2 and C4 are all associated with a very similar clinical picture. Patients typically present with recurrent pyogenic infections and/or a disease closely resembling SLE. The disease association with pyogenic microorganisms[67] presumably reflects the important role of complement in the opsonization of these bacteria for phagocytosis. It is relevant in this context that deficiency of CR3 (considered below), an important opsonic receptor on leukocytes, allows infection with a similar spectrum of bacteria. The lysis of most pyogenic bacteria by complement is probably not an important mechanism of host defence because deficiency of components of the lytic pathway of complement is not associated with an excess of pyogenic infection apart from *Neisseriae*, considered below.

The mechanism of the association of inherited deficiency of these complement proteins with SLE-like disease is not fully understood. Four complement components are inherited in the major histocompatibility complex (MHC): C4a, C4b, C2 and Factor B (Class III gene products) and are therefore closely linked to Class II gene products. It has been suggested that deficiencies of these HLA-linked complement proteins in SLE are acting as linkage markers for the true disease susceptibility genes, the Class II HLA-D region genes. However, there are three major reasons for believing that this association is truly physiological. Firstly, similar illness is associated with deficiency of a number of different complement components which are encoded in different regions of the genome. Secondly, acquired complement deficiency is itself associated with SLE-like disease. Inherited hemizygous deficiency of C1 inhibitor (hereditary angio-oedema, HAE) causes an inability to adequately regulate the activation of C1r and C1s, and this in turn leads to consumption of C4 and C2. About 2% of patients with HAE develop a lupus-like illness[68, 69]. Similarly, a small number of patients with C3 nephritic factor (C3nef) develop immune complex disease (reviewed in ref. 65). C3nef is an antibody that stabilizes the C3 convertase enzyme, C3bBb, and thereby causes uncontrolled amplification of the cleavage of C3 which cycles to completion. The third argument is that complement deficiency appears to be very rare in healthy subjects, with two exceptions discussed below. This excludes the possibilty that complement deficiency is common in patients with SLE simply because this is the population in which complement is measured, i.e. an association due to ascertainment bias.

Heidelberger[70] was the first to recognize that complement played an important role in modifying the lattice of immune complexes (reviewed in ref. 71) and this may be a mechanism whereby complement deficiency plays a role in inducing immune complex disease. The formation of large latticed immune complexes which precipitate from solution is inhibited by components of the classical pathway of complement: C1q may inhibit Fc–Fc interactions between immunoglobulins; the covalent deposition of C4 and of C3 on to components of the immune complex may alter the valency of the antigen for antibody and thereby inhibit large lattice formation[72]. In the presence of complement deficiency the normal mechanisms of disposal of immune complexes formed of self-antigens and low levels of autoantibodies may fail. These immune complexes would deposit in tissues where they could evoke inflammation, release of more autoantigen and amplification of the autoantibody response.

An alternative explanation for the link between complement deficiency and SLE may be that complement deficiency allows the establishment of chronic viral infection with secondary development of autoimmunity. *In vitro* studies with virally-infected cells have shown that viral antigens may be modulated on the surface of infected cells by antibody alone, allowing persistent infection[73]. In the presence of antibody *and* complement infected cells could be lysed[74]. It is intriguing that children with subacute sclerosing pan-encephalitis were recently reported to have a very high prevalence of partial C4 deficiency[75], suggesting that this mechanism of host defence may be important in preventing persistent measles infection in the central nervous system. However, these observations need to be confirmed.

The prevalence of both pyogenic and immune complex disease is higher amongst patients with deficiency of the C1 subcomponents or of C4 (about 80%) than amongst those with complete C2 deficiency (approximately 60%). This may be explained by the fact that C4 may function as an opsonin and that immune complex precipitation is partly inhibited by C1q and by C4, and therefore deficiencies of these proteins may have a more deleterious effect than deficiency of C2.

C4a and C4b

Before considering the association of complement deficiencies with idiopathic SLE, where in the vast majority of cases there is no overt hereditary complement deficiency, it is first necessary to consider aspects of the biology of C4. There are two isotypes of C4, both showing extensive inherited structural polymorphisms[76, 77] which include non-expressed products (C4 null alleles), encoded by closely linked genes in the MHC between the HLA-D and -B regions. Small quantities of C4 are normally deposited on erythrocytes where they may be detected as blood groups by allo-antisera. C4a is usually detected as the Rodgers blood group and C4b as Chido. There are functional differences between the two isotypes: C4b showing far greater capacity to lyse erythrocytes than C4a. The biochemical explanation for these functional differences has recently been elucidated[78, 79]. C4 and C3 both contain labile internal thio-ester bonds which upon activation of the parent molecule are enabled to form covalent linkages with adjacent amine or hydroxyl groups. C4a is efficient at binding to amine groups, forming an amide bond, whilst C4b binds more efficiently to hydroxyl bonds, forming an ester bond. Thus C4a interacts best with proteins, whilst C4b mainly attaches to carbohydrate groups which predominate on cell surfaces.

Null alleles for C4a and C4b are common amongst Caucasoid populations (approximately 35% have one or more null alleles[80]) and these commonly occur in one of two haplotypes: C4aQO, C4b1 or C4a3, C4bQO[81]; the haplotype C4aQO, C4bQO is very rare and accounts for the extreme rarity of total C4 deficiency. However, total deficiency of either C4a or C4b is fairly common (about 4% and 1% in a Caucasiod population respectively).

Idiopathic SLE and C2 and C4 null alleles

The majority of patients with SLE do not have overt inherited complement deficiency, although consumption *in vivo* of the components of the classical pathway of complement is an important feature of active disease. Partial inherited complement deficiencies may play an important role in such individuals. Thus heterozygous C2 deficiency has been associated with SLE and juvenile arthritis[82]. SLE in Caucasoid subjects has known for some time to be associated with products of the MHC and in particular with HLA-DR3 (reviewed in ref. 83). Family studies have narrowed this association to a particular haplotype, HLA-A1, -B8, -DR3. This haplotype contains a null gene (with no detectable product) for C4a and there is increasing evidence that it may be this gene that is the disease susceptibility gene for the majority of patients with SLE[84]. In Caucasoid subjects there is strong linkage disequilibrium between HLA-DR3 and C4aQO, which hinders the distinction between the relative contributions of these two genes as disease susceptibility genes. However, studies in other racial groups in which HLA-DR3 is rare may soon be expected to provide a clear answer.

Deficiency of C3 and of alternative pathway components

C3 deficiency has been described in 12 individuals[85] of whom 11 had bacterial infections (resembling the infections seen with antibody deficiency) and eight had some manifestations of immune complex disease; none of these subjects was entirely healthy. The antibody response was relatively normal in these patients, which emphasizes that complement is not necessary for the induction of antibody synthesis (see below for discussion of CR2). Inherited deficiency of Factor I (described in eight patients) and Factor H (subtotal deficiency described in two brothers) result in consumption of C3 since the amplification loop cannot be regulated[86]. Once again the disease associations are with pyogenic infections, immune complex disease and meningococcal infections[67, 85].

Deficiencies of the other components of the alternative pathway seem very rare although this may partly be because screening tests for alternative pathway function are less frequently performed. Properdin deficiency has been described in a few pedigrees associated with recurrent bacterial infections and is apparently an X-linked trait[87]. Factor B deficiency has only been described in heterozygote form[88] and Factor D deficiency in adult monozygotic twins with recurrent respiratory infections[89].

Deficiency of components of the membrane attack complex

The predominant disease association of the inherited late complement component deficiencies is infection with *Neisseriae*, mainly *N. meningitidis*. Lysis of these bacteria by the membrane attack complex is an important means of host defence, presumably because they are capable of intracellular survival. The majority of patients with late component deficiencies are ascertained by the screening of patients with recurrent meningococcal infections and the prevalence of complement deficiency, both inherited and acquired, in these individuals is remarkably high[90, 91]. In affluent Western societies, where endemic meningococcal disease has become rare, many subjects with these complement deficiencies may never be identified.

An exceptionally high prevalence of C6 deficiency has been described in the Cape coloured population of South Africa (Dr Ann Orren, personal communication). The high prevalence of this deficiency suggests that the null gene may actually have some protective effect in this population; one possibility is that the effects of endotoxic shock are mitigated in the presence of C6 deficiency.

C9 deficiency is very common in Japanese (gene frequency 0.03) and has no disease associations[92]. The deficiency of C9 in this population may not be absolute and this may explain the lack of associated disease. Meningococcal disease has been reported in one of the very few non-Japanese described with C9 deficiency[93]. An alternative explanation is that C8 may be able to cause sufficient lysis to protect against Neisserial disease. The Japanese C9-deficient patients had an average CH50 of 12 units (normal 30–50 units in this population), but less than 2% of normal antigenic C9 concentration. Once again, it is uncertain what the survival value of the C9 deficient gene may be.

A few patients with SLE-like disease and deficiency of one of the components of the membrane attack complex have been described[94-97]. The prevalence of lupus-like disease associated with C5–C8 deficiency is much lower than in patients with early component deficiencies and the mechanism of disease susceptibility is less clear. Deficiency of C5–C9 is not associated with abnormality of complement-mediated immune complex lattice modification.

COMPLEMENT RECEPTORS AND THEIR DEFICIENCIES

Introduction

Deficiency states have been described for two of the three well-defined receptors for the major fragments of C3 (complement receptors types 1, 2 and 3; CR1, CR2 and CR3). Pertinent details of these receptors are shown in Table 8.1 (reviewed in ref. 98). The majority of CR1 is located on erythrocytes in the circulation of primates. On these cells its expression is governed in normal subjects by a balanced inherited numerical polymorphism[99-101]. In addition, there is an acquired deficiency of CR1 seen on erythrocytes from patients with certain diseases, amongst which the common denominator

Table 8.1 Complement receptors for C3

Complement receptor	Ligands	Cellular distribution
CR1	C3b>C4b >iC3b C3i, C3c	erythrocytes, neutrophils monocytes, B and some T cells glomerular epithelial cells dendritic reticulum cells
CR2	iC3b, C3dg Epstein–Barr virus	B lymphocytes, epithelium of nasopharynx and cervix
CR3	iC3b, *S. cerevisiae*, *S. epidermidis*, *H. capsulatum*	monocytes, neutrophils macrophages, NK cells

appears to be the deposition of C3 on the erythrocyte surface. This deficiency is considered in detail below.

No deficiency of CR2 has so far been reported. CR2 is mainly located on B lymphocytes and preliminary evidence suggests that ligation of the receptor by immune complexes bearing C3dg or iC3b may enhance B cell activation[102]. Guinea pigs deficient in C4 or C2 show impaired antibody responses at low doses of antigen, though this impairment is overcome at conventional immunizing doses of antigens[103]. CR2 is also the Epstein–Barr virus receptor[104,105] and has been demonstrated on certain epithelia including those lining nasopharynx[106] and cervix[107]. It has recently been cloned[108] and belongs to the superfamily of structurally related proteins that contain a repeating domain of approximately 60 amino acids (see below under CR1).

CR3 is a member of another superfamily of structurally related cell surface adhesion molecules and receptors. Deficiency of CR3 and its immediate structural relatives is the cause of an important inherited immunodeficiency state that is considered below in detail.

CR1

Structure

CR1 belongs to a superfamily[109] of proteins containing a repeating domain of approximately 60 amino acids. Proteins so far shown to belong to this family include a number of complement proteins: C4 binding protein (C4bp), Factor H (FH) and CR1 (all encoded by a linked cluster of genes on chromosome 1); the 'a' regions of C2 and Factor B (encoded by genes within the major histocompatibility complex on chromosome 6); CR2[108] and decay accelerating factor (DAF). These proteins all have in common an ability to bind to C3 and C4 fragments. A number of non-complement proteins also contain this domain, including glycoprotein β2-I and IL-2 receptor which are not known to bind to C3 or C4.

CR1 is predominantly a cell surface-bound molecule and its cellular distribution is described in Table 8.1; a very small amount of free CR1 has been measured in plasma[110] and this presumably has been released from cell surfaces.

Inherited polymorphisms

CR1 shows a number of unusual genetic polymorphisms. The first is a structural polymorphism; four structural variants can be detected by their variation in molecular weight: 160 kDa, 190 kDa, 220 kDa and 250 kDa. This unprecedented variation in molecular weight is due to protein and not carbohydrate polymorphism. It will presumably be accounted for by variable duplication of the exon encoding the 60 amino acid repeating domain of which CR1 is largely composed. A restriction fragment length polymorphism (RFLP) further divides the 190 kDa variant into two subtypes. It is not yet known whether this nucleotide sequence polymorphism has a structural correlate.

A further unusual inherited polymorphism of CR1 is a numerical expression polymorphism, apparently found only on erythrocytes and not on leukocytes. Normal individuals express between 150 and 1200 molecules of CR1 per erythrocyte and this phenotype remains stable over prolonged periods. Family studies suggested that the numerical expression of CR1 was inherited. Wilson and his colleagues[101] have recently described an RFLP, detected using a cDNA probe derived from CR1, which correlates with the numerical expression of this molecule. Two variants have been detected, using the restriction enzyme Hin dIII, of sizes 6.9 kb (L) and 7.4 kb (H) and these segregate as alleles. Three phenotypes of CR1 numbers are correlated with the three possible genotypes: LL, low expression, HL, intermediate expression, and HH, high expression. There is overlap between the three phenotypic groups making it impossible to directly ascertain genotype from phenotype[101, 111]. There is some linkage disequilibrium between the H and the L allele and the structural variants of CR1, although this has not been fully elucidated[112].

Function

CR1 is an important opsonic receptor and this function is considered below. However, the majority of CR1 in the circulation of primates (in non-primates CR1 is located on platelets rather than on erythrocytes) is bound to erythrocytes where it has two main physiological functions. The first is as a cofactor to the serine esterase Factor I which cleaves C3b to sequentially iC3b and then C3dg plus C3c. Factor H functions as an alternative cofactor to CR1 for the first of these cleavage reactions; CR1 is apparently the sole cofactor for the second step[113-115]. Bacteria or immune complexes which bear iC3b are capable of binding to CR1 and CR3 on phagocytic cells; these receptors will not bind to particles bearing bound C3dg. Complete catabolism of C3 on immune complexes may help to neutralize their phlogistic potential and CR1 deficiency might therefore be predicted to have deleterious effects in diseases mediated by immune complexes.

The second physiological role of CR1 on erythrocytes appears to be in the transport of particles which bear bound C3b or iC3b from the circulation to the fixed reticuloendothelial system. Indeed CR1 was first recognized as a receptor that mediated the 'immune adherence' of alexinated trypanosomes to rodent platelets and to human erythrocytes. Recent *in vitro* studies have shown that immune complexes, after alexination, associate predominantly with erythrocytes[116]. This association is reversible: FI releases the immune complexes from CR1 as it catabolizes iC3b on the complexes to C3dg[114] which no longer has affinity for CR1. However, the physical association of alexinated particles to cellular CR1 may enable their efficient clearance from the circulation to the fixed reticuloendothelial system.

Experimental evidence in support of this idea comes from the studies of Cornacoff and his associates[117-119]. They have conducted a series of experiments on the fate of radiolabelled immune complexes injected into the circulation of baboons. These immune complexes bind to erythrocytes *in vivo* and are rapidly cleared from the circulation in the liver and spleen; immune complexes injected into decomplemented animals or immune complexes that fix complement poorly do not bind to erythrocytes and are cleared more rapidly from the ciculation, some to sites outside the reticuloendothelial system where they may cause inflammation. We have recently studied the fate of artificial iodinated immune complexes in humans and found that they bind to erythrocytes *in vivo* in a complement-dependent manner and that these complexes are cleared more rapidly if CR1 numbers are low and in patients with hypocomplementaemia[119a].

Deficiency

A reduction of erythrocyte CR1 numerical expression has been found in a number of diseases which include SLE[99, 100, 120-123], autoimmune haemolytic anaemias, paroxysmal nocturnal haemoglobinuria[124] and AIDS[125]. A common feature of the first three of these diseases is the presence of complement activation on or in close vicinity to the erythrocyte membrane. Although there has been some dispute as to whether the low levels of erythrocyte CR1 seen in patients with SLE are acquired or inherited, a number of lines of evidence show that it is mainly an acquired abnormality. Thus CR1 levels in patients correlate with disease activity[121, 123, 126] and with the amount of C3dg bound to the erythrocyte surface[123]. Furthermore CR1 is lost from erythrocytes transfused into patients with active disease[123a] and family studies have shown patients with SLE with much lower levels of CR1 than their consanguineous relatives[100]. Finally, using the RFLP correlating with numerical expression of CR1 on erythrocytes, we have shown that the allele linked to low expression of erythrocyte CR1 is not a disease susceptibility gene for SLE[111].

CR3, LFA-1, p150, 95

Structure

These molecules share a common β chain, encoded on chromosome 21, and have individual α chains (for LFA-1 on chromosome 16)[127]. There is sequence homology between the NH2-terminal portions of CR3 and LFA-1[128] and intriguingly between these molecules and an Arg-Gly-Asp receptor, the vitronectin receptor[129]. This latter receptor is a member of a group of cell surface receptors that includes the fibronectin receptor and the GpIIb/IIIa glycoprotein of platelets. Cosgrove and colleagues[130] have published a preliminary description of a genomic clone (of size 20 kb) apparently encoding the α chain of CR3, LFA-1 and glycoprotein IIb/IIIa. However, the α chain of the murine homologue of CR3 has recently been cloned[131] and its large size (11.9 kb) is not compatible with the data of Cosgrove and colleagues, unless the organization of murine and human DNA encoding these molecules is very different.

Function

Functional characterization of this family of molecules has shown them to have receptor activities and also to be important in intercellular adhesion.

CR3 binds diverse ligands in a cation-dependent manner; such as iC3b, zymosan[132], and the lipid A portion of lipopolysaccharide[133]. This diverse binding spectrum has a precedent in the structurally unrelated molecule, bovine conglutinin, which similarly binds to iC3b and to zymosan in a cation-dependent manner[134]. Wright and colleagues[133] have shown that LFA-1 and p 150,95 also bind to bacterial lipopolysaccharides, and will therefore bind to organisms such as smooth *E. coli* and *H. capsulatum*. The ingestion of *S. epidermidis* by normal neutrophils could be inhibited by antibodies to the α chains of LFA-1 or CR3 or by anti-β chain[135]. The ligands for LFA-1 and for p 150, 95 have not been clearly established. There is some evidence that p 150, 95 may bind to iC3b [136] and thus may be another complement receptor.

The relative contributions of CR3, LFA-1, and p 150,95 to neutrophil adhesiveness have recently been assessed *in vitro* using monoclonal antibodies as specific inhibitors[137]; the ranking was CR3 > p 150,95 > LFA-1. In contrast, homotypic adhesiveness of lymphocytes appears to be governed exclusively by LFA-1[138-140] and that of activated U937 cells (a macrophage-like line) by p 150,95[141].

CR1 and CR3 as opsonic receptors

Both CR1 and CR3 function as important opsonic receptors on phagocytic cells of myeloid origin. It has only recently been appreciated that the function of both of these receptors is precisely and co-ordinately regulated. Kay and colleagues[142] showed enhancement of C3b-mediated rosetting to leukocytes by chemotactic agents; this enhancement can partially be explained by an increase in the numerical expression of both CR1[143] and CR3[144], though not entirely[145]. The increased surface expression of both these receptors following stimulation is rapid and not dependent on protein synthesis. Distinct intracellular pools exist for these molecules; CR3 is found in the specific granules of neutrophils[146-148] whilst CR1 is located in a membrane-associated pool. Chemotactic stimuli also increase the surface expression of p 150,95[149] but not of LFA-1.

The ligand-binding activity and consequence of receptor ligation are also regulated. Prolonged incubation of neutrophils and monocytes with phorbol myristal acetate (PMA) abolishes the ability of CR1 and CR3 to bind their respective ligands, as does interferon-γ[150, 151]. This is not accomplished by loss of cell surface receptors. In contrast, CR1 and CR3 require activation signals in order to mediate phagocytosis; such signals include the ligation of other cell surface receptors for laminin[152] or fibronectin[153] or brief exposure to PMA[154]. This receptor activation event may be accomplished by receptor phosphorylation.

Deficiency of CR3, LFA-1 and p 150,95

An immunodeficiency syndrome caused by an inherited deficiency of a major family of cellular receptors and adhesion molecules has been extensively characterized during the last few years (reviewed in ref. 155). Initial clinical reports described children with a syndrome comprising delayed separation of the umbilical cord, cutaneous and deep-seated infections, gingivitis with loss of teeth and abnormal paper-thin scarring of skin[156-166]. Typical infecting organisms include *P. pyocyaneus*, *E. coli*, *K. aeruginosa* and *S. aureus*. Investigation of these children showed peripheral blood neutrophilia but poor migration of neutrophils into sites of infection and into skin windows, studies that were interpreted to show that the underlying defect in this disease was one of neutrophil malfunction.

The next major advance in elucidating the cause of this disease was the discovery that a major neutrophil surface glycoprotein was missing in affected children[158, 161, 162, 166, 167]. However the heterogenous severity of expression of the syndrome[168], coupled with differences in the estimated molecular weight of the missing protein (resolved by Anderson and colleagues, ref. 169) led to confusion about the classification of these children. With the development of many monoclonal antibodies to leukocyte surface antigens it was found that the deficient glycoprotein was a molecule (initially defined by the antibodies OKM1[170], Mol[171] and MN41[135], normally located on monocytes and neutrophils. This finding has allowed the easy, specific identification of affected children and the recognition that the severity of the clinical syndrome is related to the degree of deficiency of the family of molecules[168].

The biochemical characterization of the lesion has largely been due to Springer and his colleagues, who have shown that a whole family of three cell surface molecules CR3, LFA-1 and p150,95[172], defined initially by mono-clonal antibodies, is missing in these patients.

Biosynthetic studies have shown that the defect in patients appears to reside at the level of synthesis of the β chain[173]. The nature of the genetic lesion(s) is not yet clear. The syndrome has been described in several ethnic groups, the sex ratio of sufferers is approximately equal and some parents have been found to show reduced expression of the family of molecules. These observations imply that the disease is inherited as an autosomal recessive condition and that the abnormal gene may be only moderately rare.

The discovery of these children has made it possible to determine the physiological function *in vivo* of this family of molecules. The major features of disease appear to be secondary to neutrophil dysfunction and the clinical features are similar to other inherited disorders of neutrophils. With a single exception[174], antibody responses have been normal and major viral infections have not been a clinical problem. Similarly, delayed-type hypersensitivity appears normal. *In vitro* studies of leukocytes from affected patients have shown severely depressed natural killer cell activity and reduced antibody-dependent cytotoxicity[175]. The clinical effect of these latter abnormalities is not so far apparent.

Early studies of neutrophils from these patients showed that they had reduced spreading and anchoring on plastic surfaces and on fibronectin- and endotoxin-coated surfaces. Of interest were observations that when patient neutrophils were mixed with normal neutrophils they would both adhere and aggregate normally[169, 176]; these observations show that it is not an adherence 'receptor' that is deficient. Anderson and colleagues[169] performed extensive experiments which showed impaired adherence- and adhesion-dependent cellular functions; these included reduced adherence and spreading on surfaces, orientation in chemotactic gradients, aggregation and phagocytosis. Adherence-independent functions were all normal and included shape changes, f-met-leu-phe-binding and oxygen radical generation to soluble stimuli. Neutrophils showed reduced binding of latex-coated beads but normal redistribution of adhesion sites to the cell uropod following stimulation with a chemotactic agent.

The findings of Arnaout and colleagues[167] suggested that both Fc- and C3b-receptor activity were abnormal in a patient with deficiency of 'gp 150'. However, a number of observations hindered the discovery that the molecule which was missing from patients' cells was actually a receptor for complement. Initial studies showed that rosetting of IgG-[158] and C3b-bearing particles was normal[158, 167]. It was also found in some studies that phagocytosis of IgG-bearing particles was reduced[167, 170] and that this effect could be induced by a monoclonal antibody (Mo-1) to the missing neutrophil glycoprotein. However, Ross showed that the conditions for the performance of C3-dependent rosettes are critical. In order to demonstrate a deficiency of CR3-mediated rosetting it was necessary to inhibit neutrophil CR1 using a polyclonal antibody[135, 171, 177]. Similarly, the density of the ligand used in rosetting studies significantly influences the findings. Abnormal ingestion of IgG-coated particles is seen at low IgG densities[132]. This is presumably because CR3 plays a co-operative role in phagocytosis via its adhesive properties.

The impaired ability of monocytes and neutrophils to bind to both opsonized and to unopsonized microorganisms (discussed above) probably explains the spectrum of infections seen in these patients.

CONCLUSIONS

Fascinating insights into the complex biology and biochemistry of phagocytic cells and the complement system are emerging through detailed investigations into the pathophysiology of rare and varied experiments of nature. An important role for these systems of host defence in the control of infections has been demonstrated by studying those unfortunate individuals with hereditary protein deficiencies affecting phagocyte and complement function. Recurrent infections with *Neisseriae* or pyogenic bacteria suggests the presence of an inherited immunodeficiency syndrome. Full investigation of these individuals is worthwhile and may enable correct prophylactic measures to be taken. In cases where inherited complement deficiency is associated with immune complex disease, it may be that repletion of complement may have a therapeutic role. However this is only just becoming technically feasible.

ACKNOWLEDGEMENTS

We would like to thank the Wellcome Trust, the Medical Research Council and the Arthritis and Rheumatism Council for support.

References

1. White, C. J. and Gallin, J. I. (1986). Phagocyte defects, *Clin. Immunol. Immunopathol.*, **40** 50-61
2. Klebanoff, S. J. and Clark, R. A. (1978). In *The Neutrophil*. Ch. 10. (Amsterdam: North Holland)
3. Gallin, J. I. and Fauci, A. S. (eds.) (1983). *Advances in Host Defence Mechanisms*. Vol. 3. (New York: Raven Press)
4. Johnston, R. B. and Newman, S. L. (1977). Chronic granulomatous disease. *Ped. Clin. N. Am.*, **24**, 365-76
5. Quie, P. G., White, J. G., Holmes, B. and Good, R. A. (1967). *In vitro* bactericidal capacity of human polymorphonuclear leukocytes: diminished activity in chronic granulomatous disease of childhood. *J. Clin. Invest.*, **46**, 668-79
6. Thompson, E. N. and Soothill, J. F. (1970). Chronic granulomatous disease: qualitative clinicopathological relationships. *Arch. Dis. Child.*, **45**, 24-32
7. Segal, A. W. and Coade, S. (1978). Kinetics of oxygen consumption by phagocytosing human neutrophils. *Biochem. Biophys. Res. Commun.*, **84**, 611-17
8. Baldridge, C. W. and Gerard, R. W. (1933). The extra respiration of phagocytosis. *Am. J. Physiol.*, **103**, 235-6
9. Sbarra, A. J. and Karnovsky, M. L. (1959). The biochemical basis of phagocytosis. 1. Metabolic changes during the ingestion of particles by polymorphonuclear leukocytes. *J. Biol. Chem.*, **234**, 1355-62
10. Selvaraj, R. J. and Sbarra, A. J. (1966). Relationship of glycolytic and oxidative metabolism to particle entry and destruction in phagocytosing cells. *Nature (London)*, **211**, 1272-6
11. Mandell, G. L. (1974). Bactericidal activity of aerobic and anaerobic polymorphonuclear neutrophils. *Infect. Immunol.*, **9**, 337-41
12. Holmes, B., Page, A. R. and Good, R. A. (1967). Studies of the metabolic activity of leukocytes from patients with a genetic abnormality of phagocyte function. *J. Clin. Invest.*, **46**, 1422-32
13. Sternholm, R. and Manak, R. C. (1970). Carbohydrate metabolism in leukocytes. XIV. Regulation of pentose cycle activity and glycogen metabolism during phagocytosis. *J. Reticuloendoth. Soc.*, **8**, 550-60
14. Segal, A. W. and Jones, O. T. G. (1978). Novel cytochrome b system in phagocytic vacuoles from human granulocytes. *Nature (London)*, **276**, 515-17
15. Cross, A. R., Jones, O. T. G., Harper A. M. and Segal, A. W. (1981). Oxidation-reduction properties of the cytochrome b found in the plasma-membrane fraction of human neutrophils. A possible oxidase in the respiratory burst. *Biochem. J.*, **194**, 599-606
16. Segal, A. W. and Jones, O. T. G. (1979). The subcellular distribution and some properties of the cytochrome b component of the microbicidal oxidase system of human neutrophils. *Biochem. J.*, **182**, 181-8
17. Garcia, R. C. and Segal, A. W. (1984). Changes in the subcellular distribution of the cytochrome b-245 on stimulation of human neutrophils. *Biochem. J.*, **219**, 233-42
18. Segal, A. W. and Jones, O. T. G. (1980). Rapid incorporation of the human neutrophil plasma membrane cytochrome b into phagocytic vacuoles. *Biochem. Biophys. Res. Commun.*, **92**, 710-15
19. Cross, A. R., Higson, F. K., Jones, O. T. G., Harper, A. M. and Segal, A. W. (1982). The enzymic reduction and kinetics of oxidation of cytochrome b-245 of neutrophils. *Biochem. J.*, **204**, 479-85
20. Cross, A. R., Parkinson, J. F. and Jones, O. T. G. (1985). Mechanism of the superoxide producing oxidase of neutrophils is necessary for the fast reduction of cytochrome b-245 by NADPH. *Biochem. J.*, **226**, 881-4
21. Segal, A. W. (1988). Absence of the two subunits of cytochrome b-245 from neutrophils in X-linked chronic granulomatous disease. *Nature*, In press
22. Harper, A. M., Chaplin, M. F. and Segal, A. W. (1985). Cytochrome b-245 from human neutrophils is a glycoprotein. *Biochem. J.*, **227**, 783-8
23. Poole, R. K. (1983). Bacterial cytochrome oxidases. A structurally and functionally diverse group of electron-transfer proteins. *Biochim. Biophys. Acta*, **726**, 205-43

24. Cross, A. R., Jones, O. T. G., Garcia, R. and Segal, A. W. (1982). The association of FAD with the cytochrome b-245 of human neutrophils. *Biochem. J.*, **208**, 759–63
25. Light, D. R., Walsh, C., O'Callaghan, A. M., Goetzl, E. J. and Tauber, A. I. (1981). Characteristics of the cofactor requirements for the superoxide-generating NADPH oxidase of human polymorphonuclear leukocytes. *Biochemistry*, **20**, 1468–76
26. Millard, J. A., Gerard, K. W. and Schneider, D. L. (1979). The isolation from rat peritoneal leukocytes of plasma membrane enriched in alkaline phosphatase and a b-type cytochrome. *Biochem. Biophys. Res. Commun.*, **90**, 312–19
27. Crawford, D. R. and Schneider, D. L. (1982). Identification of ubiquinone 50 in human neutrophils and its role in microbicidal events. *J. Biol. Chem.*, **257**, 6662–8
28. Cunningham, C. C., De Chatelet, L. R., Spach, P. I., Parce, J. W., Thomas, M. J., Lees, C. J. and Shirley, P. S. (1982). Identification and quantitation of electron transport components in human polymorphonuclear neutrophils. *Biochim. Biophys. Acta*, **682**, 430–35
29. Cross, A. R., Jones, O. T. G., Garcia, R. C. and Segal, A. W. (1983). The subcellular localization of ubiquinone in human neutrophils. *Biochem. J.*, **216**, 765–8
30. Hitzig, W. H. and Seger, R. A. (1983). Chronic granulomatous disease, a heterogenous syndrome. *Hum. Genet.*, **64**, 207–15
31. Hamers, M. N., de Boer, M., Meerhof, L. J., Weening, R. S. and Roos, D. (1988). Complementation in monocyte hybrids revealing genetic heterogeneity in chronic granulomatous disease. *Nature (London)*, In press
32. Segal, A. W., Cross, A. R., Garcia, R. C., Borregaard, N., Valerius, N. H., Soothill, J. F. and Jones, O. T. G. (1983). Absence of cytochrome b-245 in chronic granulomatous disease. A multicentre European evaluation of its incidence and relevance. *N. Engl. J. Med.*, **308**, 245–51
33. Ohno, Y., Buescher, E. S., Roberts, R., Metcalf, J. A. and Gallin, J. (1986). Reevaultion of cytochrome b and flavin adenine dinucleotide in neutrophils from patients with chronic granulomatous disease and description of a family with probable autosomal recessive inheritance of cytochrome b deficiency. *Blood*, **67**, 1132–8
34. Franke, U., Ochs, H. D., de Martinville, B. *et al.* (1985). Minoe Xp 21 chromosome deletion in a malt associated with expression of Duchenne muscular dystropy, chronic gravulomators disease, retinits pigmentosa and McLeod syndrome. *Am. J. Hum. Genet.*, **37**, 250–67
35. Royer-Pokora, B. *et al.* (1986). Cloning the gene for an inherited human disorder – chronic granulomatous disease – on the basis of its chromosomal location. *Nature*, **322**, 32–8
36. Segal, A. W. and Jones, O. T. G. (1980). Absence of cytochrome b reduction in stimulated neutrophils from both female and male patients with chronic granulomatous disease. *FEBS Letts.*, **110**, 111–14
37. Gennaro, R., Florio, C. and Romeo, N. (1985). Activation of protein kinase C in neutrophil cytoplasts. Localization of protein substrates and possible relationship with stimulus-response coupling. *FEBS Letts.*, **180**, 185–90
38. Berridge, M. J. (1984). Inositol triphosphate and diacylglycerol as second messengers. *Biochem. J.*, **220**, 345–60
39. Segal, A. W., Heyworth, P. G., Cockroft, S. and Barrowman, M. M. (1985). Stimulated neutrophils from patients with autosomal recessive chronic granulomatous disease fail to phosphorylate a M,44,000 kDa protein. *Nature (London)*. **316**, 547–9
40. Gray, G. R. *et al.* (1973). Neutrophil dysfunction, chronic granulomatous disease and nonspherocytic haemolytic anaemia caused by complete deficiency of glucose-6-phosphate dehydrogenase. *Lancet*, **2**, 530–4
41. Harvath, L. and Anderson, B. R. (1979). Defective initiation of oxidative metabolism in polymorphonuclear leukocytes. *N. Engl. J. Med.*, **300**, 1130–5
42. Segal, A. W., Geisow, M., Garcia, R., Harper, A. and Miller, R. (1981). The respiratory burst of phagocytic cells is associated with a rise in vacuolar pH. *Nature*, **290**, 406–9
43. Babior, B. M., Kipnes, R. S. and Curnutte, J. T. (1973). The production by leukocytes of superoxide, a potential bactericidal agent. *J. Clin. Invest.*, **52**, 741–4
44. Iyer, G. Y. N., Islam, D. M. F. and Quastel, J. H. (1961). Biochemical aspects of phagocytosis. *Nature*, **192**, 535–41
45. Roos, D., Voetman, A. A. and Meerhof, L. J. (1983). Functional activity of enucleated human polymorphonuclear leukocytes. *J. Cell Biol.*, **97**, 368–77

46. Ambruso, D. R. and Johnston, R. B. (1981). Lactoferrin enhances hydroxyl radical production by human neutrophils, neutrophil particulate fractions and an enzymic generating system. *J. Clin. Invest.*, **67**, 352

47. Gutteridge, J. M., Paterson, S. K., Segal, A. W. and Halliwell, B. (1981). Inhibition of lipid peroxidation by the iron-binding protein lactoferrin. *Biochem. J.*, **199**, 259-61

48. Klebanoff, S. J. (1975). Antimicrobial mechanisms in neutrophilic polymorphonuclear leukocytes. *Semin. Hematol.*, **12**, 117-42

49. Winterbourn, C. C., Garcia, R. C. and Segal, A. W. (1985). Production of the superoxide adduct of myeloperoxidase (compound 111) by stimulated human neutrophils, and its reactivity with hydrogen peroxide and chloride. *Biochem. J.*, **288**, 583-92

50. Odeberg, H. and Olsson, I. (1975). Antibacterial activity of cationic proteins from human granulocytes. *J. Clin. Invest.*, **56**, 1118-24

51. Barrett, A. J. (1969). Properties of lysosomal enzymes. In Dingle, J. T. and Fell, H. B. (eds.) *Lysosomes in Biology and Pathology*. Vol. 2, p. 244. (Amsterdam: North Holland)

52. Jacques, Y. V. and Bainton, D. F. (1978). Changes in pH within the phagocytic vacuoles of human neutrophils and monocytes. *Lab. Invest.*, **39**, 179-85

53. Cech, P. and Lehrer, R. I. (1984). Phagolysosomal pH of human neutrophils. *Blood*, **63**, 88-95

54. Gabig, T. G., Lefker, B. A., Ossanna, P. J. and Weiss, S. J. (1984). Proton stoichiometry associated with human neutrophil respiratory-burst reactions. *J. Biol. Chem.*, **259**, 13166-71

55. Segal, A. W., Harper, A. M., Garcia, R. C. and Merzbach, D. (1982). The action of cells from patients with chronic granulomatous disease on *Staphylococcus aureus*. *J. Med. Microbiol.*, **15**, 441-9

56. Klebanoff, S. J. and Clark, R. A. (1978). The neutrophil. Function and clinical disorders. pp. 38-42. (Amsterdam, New York: North-Holland)

57. Landing, B. H. and Shirkey, H. S. (1957). A syndrome of recurrent infection and infiltration of viscera by pigmented lipid histiocytes. *Pediatrics*, **20**, 431-8

58. Newburger, P. E., Cohen, H. J., Rothchild, S. B. *et al.* (1979). Prenatal diagnosis of chronic granulomatous disease. *N. Engl. J. Med.*, **300**, 181-3

59. Segal, A. W. and Peters, T. J. (1975). The nylon column dye test: a possible screening test of phagocytic function. *Clin. Sci. Mol. Med.*, **49**, 591-6

60. Trush, M. A., Wilson, M. E. and Van Dyke, K. (1978). The generation of chemiluminescence (CL) by phagocytic cells. *Meth. Enzymol.*, **57**, 462

61. Babior, B. M. and Cohen, H. J. (1981). Measurement of neutrophil function: phagocytosis, degranulation, the respiratory burst and bacterial killing. In Cline, M. J. (ed.), *Methods in Hematology*, Vol. 3, pp. 1-38. (London: Churchill Livingstone)

62. Segal, A. W., Harper, A. M., Cross, A. R. and Jones, O. T. G. (1988). Purification and properties of cytochrome b-245. *Meth. Enzymol.*, in press

63. Rausch, P. G., Pryzwansky K. B. and Spitznagel, J. K. (1978). Immunocytochemical identification of azurophilic and specific granule markers in giant granules of Chediak-Higashi neutrophils. *N. Engl. J. Med.*, **298**, 693-8

64. Pollard, H. B., Shindo, H., Creutz, C. E., Pazoles, C. J. and Cohen, J. S. (1979). Internal pH and state of ATP in adrenergic chromaffin granules determined by ^{31}P nuclear magnetic resonance spectroscopy. *J. Biol. Chem.*, **254**, 1170-7

65. Hobart, M. J., Walport, M. J. and Lachmann, P. J. (1984). Complement polymorphism and disease. *Clin. Immunol. All*, **4**, 647-64

66. Lachmann, P. J. (1984). Inherited complement deficiencies. *Philos. Trans. R. Soc. Lond. (Biol.)*, **306**, 419-30

67. Ross, S. C. and Densen, P. (1984). Complement deficiency states and infection. *Medicine*, **62**, 243-73

68. Donaldson, V. H., Hess, E. V. and McAdam, A. J. (1977). Lupus erythematosus-like syndrome in three unrelated women with hereditary angioneurotic edema. *Ann. Intern. Med.*, **86**, 312-13

69. Brickman, C. M., Tsokos, G. C., Balow, J. E., Lawley, T. J., Santaella, M., Hammer, C. H. and Frank, M. M. (1986). Immunoregulatory disorders associated with hereditary angioedema. 1. Clinical manifestations of autoimmune disease. *J. Allergy Clin. Immunol.*, **77**, 749-57 .

70. Heidelberger, M. (1941). Quantitative chemical studies on complement or alexin. *J. Exp.*

Med., **73**, 681-94

71. Schifferli, J. A., Ng, Y. C. and Peters, D. K. (1986). The role of complement and its receptor in the elimination of immune complexes. *N. Engl. J. Med.*, **315**, 488-95

72. Lachmann, P. J. and Walport, M. J. (1988). Deficiency of the effector mechanisms of the immune response and autoimmunity. In Whelan, J. (ed.) *Autoimmunity and Autoimmune Disease* (Ciba Foundation Symposium 129). (Chichester: Wiley) in press

73. Joseph, B. S. and Oldstone, M. B. A. (1974). Antibody-induced redistribution of measles virus antigen on the cell surface. *J. Immunol.*, **113**, 1205-11

74. Gorman, N. T. and Lachmann, P. J. (1982). *In vitro* modulation of viral cell surface glycoproteins by anti-viral antibody in the presence of complement. *Clin. Exp. Immunol.*, **50**, 507-14

75. Rittner, C., Meier, E. M. M., Stradmann, B., Giles, C. M., Kochling, R., Mollenhauer, E. and Kretch, H. W. (1984). Partial C4 deficiency in subacute sclerosing panencephalitis. *Immunogenetics*, **20**, 407-15

76. Mauff, G., Alper, C. A., Awdeh, Z., Batchelor, J. R., Bertrams, J., Bruun-Peterson, G., Dawkins, R. L., Demant, P., Edwards, J., Grosse-Wilde, H., Hauptmann, G., Klouda, P., Lamm, L., Mollenhauer, E., Nerl, C., Olaisen, B., O'Neill, G., Rittner, C., Roos, M. H., Skanes, V., Teisberg, P. and Wells, L. (1983). Statement on the nomenclature of human C4 allotypes. *Immunobiology*, **164**, 184-91

77. Yu, C. T., Belt, K. T., Giles, C. M., Campbell, R. D. and Porter, R. R. (1986). Structural basis of the polymorphism of human complement components C4A and C4B: gene size, reactivity and antigenicity. *EMBO J.*, **5**, 2873-81

78. Law, S. K. A., Dodds, A. W. and Porter, R. R. (1984). A comparison of the properties of two classes, C4A and C4B, of the complement component C4. *EMBO J.*, **3**, 1819-23

79. Isenman, D. and Young, J. R. (1984). The molecular basis for the differences in immune hemolysis activity of the Chido and Rodgers isotypes of human complement component C4. *J. Immunol.*, **132**, 3019-27

80. Hauptman, G., Goetz, J., Uring-Lambert, B. and Grosshans, E. (1986). Component deficiencies. 2. The fourth component. *Progr. Allergy*, **39**, 232-49

81. Alper, C. A., Raum, D., Karp, C., Awdeh, Z. L. and Yunis, E. J. (1983). Serum complement supergenes of the major histocompatibility complex in man (complotypes). *Vox Sang.*, **45**, 62-7

82. Glass, D., Raum, D., Gibson, D., Stillman, J. S. and Schur, P. M. (1976). Inherited deficiency of the second component of complement. *J. Clin. Invest.*, **58**, 853-61

83. Walport, M. J., Fielder, A. H. L. and Batchelor, J. R. (1984). Genetics of systemic lupus erythematosus. In Panayi, G. and David, C. (eds.) *Clinical Immunology*. 1. *Immunogenetics*. pp. 157-76. (Sevenoaks, Kent: Butterworth)

84. Fielder, A. H. L., Walport, M. J., Batchelor, J. R., Rynes, R. I., Black, C. M., Dodi, I. A. and Hughes, G. R. V. (1983). Family study of the major histocompatibility complex in patients with systemic lupus erythematosus: importance of null alleles of C4A and C4B in determining disease susceptibility. *Br. Med. J.*, **266**, 425-8

85. Schifferli, J. A. and Peters, D. K. (1983). Complement, the immune-complex lattice and the pathophysiology of complement-deficiency syndrome. *Lancet*, **2**, 957-9

86. Lachmann, P. J. (1988). Deficiencies of Factor I and Factor H. In Rother, K. and Till, G. (eds.) *The Complement System*. (Springer-Verlag) In press

87. Sjoholm, A. G., Braconier, J.-H. and Soderstrom, C. (1982). Properdin deficiency in a family with fulminant meningococcal infections. *Clin. Exp. Immunol*, **50**, 291-7

88. Mauff, G., Federman, G. and Hauptmann, G. (1980). A haemolytically inactive gene product of factor B. *Immunobiology*, **158**, 96-100

89. Hannecke, C., Kluin-Nelemans, van Velzen-Blad, H., van Helden, H. P. T. and Daha, M. R. (1984). Functional deficiency of complement factor D in a monozygous twin. *Clin. Exp. Immunol.*, **58**, 724-30

90. Merino, J., Rodriguez-Valverde, V., Lamelas, J. A., Riestra, J. L. and Casanueva, B. (1983). Prevalence of deficits of complement components in patients with recurrent meningococcal infections. *J. Infect. Dis.*, **148**, 331

91. Ellison, R. T., Kohler, P. F., Curd, J. G., Judson, F. N. and Reller, L. B. (1983). Prevalence of congenital or acquired complement deficiency in patients with sporadic meningococcal disease. *N. Engl. J. Med.*, **308**, 913-16

92. Inai, S., Kitamura, H., Hiramatsu, S. and Nagaki, K. (1979). Deficiency of the ninth component of complement in man. *J. Clin. Lab. Immunol.*, **2**, 85–7

93. Fine, D. P., Gewurz, H., Griffiss, M. and Lint, T. F. (1983). Meningococcal meningitis in a woman with inherited deficiency of the ninth component of complement. *Clin. Immunol. Immunopathol.*, **28**, 413–17

94. Rosenfield, S. I., Kelly, M. E. and Leddy, J. P. (1976). Hereditary deficiency of the fifth component in man. *J. Clin. Invest.*, **57**, 1626–43

95. Jasin, H. E. (1977). Absence of the eighth component of complement in association with systemic lupus erythematosus-like disease. *J. Clin. Invest.*, **60**, 709–15

96. Zeitz, H. J., Miller, G. W., Lint, T. F., Ali, M. A. and Gewurz, H. (1981). Deficiency of C7 with systemic lupus erythematosus. Solubilization of immune complexes in complement deficient sera. *Arthritis Rheum.*, **24**, 87–93

97. Pickering, R. J., Rynes, R. I., Locascio, N., Monahan, J. B. and Sodetz, J. M. (1982). Identification of the alpha-gamma subunit of the eighth component of complement (C8) in a patient with systemic lupus erythematosus and absent C8 activity: patients and family studies. *Clin. Immunol. Immunopathol.*, **23**, 323–4

98. Ross, G. D. and Medof, M. E. (1985). Membrane complement receptors specific for bound fragments of C3. *Adv. Immunol.*, **37**, 217–67

99. Wilson, J. G., Wong, W. W., Schur, P. H. and Fearon, D. T. (1982). Mode of inheritance of decreased C3b receptors on erythrocytes of patients with systemic lupus erythematosus. *N. Engl. J. Med.*, **307**, 981–6

100. Walport, M. J., Ross, G. D., Mackworth-Young, C., Watson, J. V., Hogg, N. and Lachmann, P. J. (1985). Family studies of erythrocyte complement receptor type I levels: reduced levels in patients with SLE are acquired, not inherited. *Clin. Exp. Immunol.*, **59**, 547–54

101. Wilson, J. G., Murphy, E. E., Wong, W. W., Klickstein, L. B., Weis, J. M. and Fearon, D. T. (1986). Identification of a restriction fragment length polymorphism by a CRl cDNA that correlates with the number of CRl on erythrocytes. *J. Exp. Med.*, **315**, 488–95

102. Melchers, F. A., Erdei, T. and Dierich, M. P. (1985). Growth control of activated, synchronized murine B cells by the C3d fragment of human complement. *Nature*, **317**, 264–7

103. Bottger, E. C., Hoffmann, T., Hadding, U. and Bitter-Suermann, D. (1985) Influence of genetically inherited complement deficiencies on humoral immune response in guinea pigs. *J. Immunol.*, **135**, 4100–7

104. Fingeroth, J. D., Weiss, J. J., Tedder, T. F., Strominger, J. L., Biro, P. A. and Fearon, D. T. (1984). Epstein–Barr virus receptor of human B lymphocytes is the C3d receptor, CR2. *Proc. Natl. Acad. Sci. (USA)*, **81**, 4510–14

105. Nemerow, G., Wolfert, R., McNaughton, M. E. and Cooper, N. R. (1985). Identification and characterization of the Epstein–Barr virus receptor on human B lymphocytes and its relationship to the C3d complement receptor (CR2). *J. Virol.*, **55**, 347–51

106. Young, L. S., Clark, D., Sixbey, J. W. and Rickinson, A. B. (1986). Epstein–Barr virus receptors on human pharyngeal epithelia. *Lancet*, **1**, 240–2

107. Sixbey, J. W., Davis, D. S., Young, L. S., Hutt-Fletcher, L., Tedder, T. F. and Rickinson, A. B. (1986). Human epithelial cell expression of an Epstein–Barr virus receptor. *Clin. Res.*, **34**, 533A (abstract)

108. Weis, J. J., Fearon, D. T., Klickstein, L. B., Wong, W. W., Richards, S. A., De Bruyn Kops, A., Smith, H. A. and Weis, J. M. (1986). Identification of a partial cDNA clone for the C3d/Epstein–Barr virus receptor of human B lymphocytes: homology with the receptor for fragments C3b and C4b of the third and fourth components of complement. *Proc. Natl. Acad. Sci. (USA)*, **83**, 5639–43

109. Holers, V. M., Cole, J. L., Lublin, D. M., Seya, T. and Atkinson, J. P. (1985). Human C3b- and C4b-regulatory proteins: a new multi-gene family. *Immunol. Today*, **6**, 188–92

110. Yoon, S. M. and Fearon, D. T. (1985). Characterization of a soluble form of the C3b/C4b receptor (CRl) in human plasma. *J. Immunol.*, **134**, 3332–8

111. Moldenhauer, F., David, J., Fielder, A. H. L., Lachmann, P. J. and Walport, M. J. (1988). Inherited deficiency of erythrocyte complement receptor type I does not cause disease susceptibility to SLE. *Arthritis Rheum.*, in press

112. Wong, W. W., Kennedy, C. A., Bonaccio, E. T., Wilson, J. G., Klickstein, L. B., Weis, J.

H. and Fearon, D. T. (1986). Analysis of multiple restriction fragment length polymorphisms of the gene for the human complement receptor type 1. *J. Exp. Med.*, **164**, 1531–46

113. Ross, G. D., Lambris, J. D., Cain, J. A. and Newman, S. L. (1982). Generation of three different fragments of bound C3 with purified factor I or serum. I. Requirements for factor H vs CR1 cofactor activity. *J. Immunol.*, **129**, 2051–60

114. Medof, M. E., Iida, K., Mold, C. and Nussenzweig, V. (1982). Unique role of the complement receptor CR1 in the degradation of C3b associated with immune complexes. *J. Exp. Med.*, **156**, 1739–54

115. Medicus, R. G., Melamed, J. and Arnaout, M. A. (1983). Role of human factor I and C3b receptor in the cleavage of surface-bound C3bi molecules. *Eur. J. Immunol.*, **13**, 465–70

116. Medof, M. E. and Oger, J. J.-F. (1982). Competition for immune complexes by red cells in human blood. *J. Clin. Lab. Immunol.*, **7**, 7–13

117. Cornacoff, J. B., Hebert, L. A., Smead, W. L., Van Aman, M. E., Birmingham, D. J. and Waxman, F. J. (1983). Primate erythrocyte-immune complex-clearing mechanism. *J. Clin. Invest.*, **71**, 236–47

118. Waxman, F. J., Herbert, L. A., Cornacoff, J. B., Van Aman, M. E., Smead, W. L., Kraut, E. M., Birmingham, D. J. and Taquiam, J. M. (1984). Complement depletion accelerates the clearance of immune complexes from the circulation of primates. *J. Clin. Invest*, **74**, 1329–40

119. Waxman, F. J., Herbert, L. A., Cosio, F. G., Smead, W. L., Van Aman, M. E., Taquiam, J. M. and Birmingham, D. J. (1986). Differential binding of immunoglobulin A and immunoglobulin G1 immune complexes to primate erythrocytes *in vivo*. *J. Clin. Invest.*, **77**, 82–9

119a. Schifferli, J. A., Ng, Y.C., Estreichee, J., Walport, M. J. (1988). The clearance of tetanus toxoid/anti-tetanus toxoid immune complexes from the circulation of humans. *J. Immunol.*, **140**, No.3

120. Miyakawa, Y., Yamada, A., Kosaka, K., Tsuda, F., Kosugi, E. and Mayumi, M. (1981). Defective immune-adherence (C3b) receptor on erythrocytes from patients with systemic lupus erythematosus. *Lancet*, **2**, 493–7

121. Iida, K., Mornaghi, R. and Nussenzweig, V. (1982). Complement receptor (CR1) deficiency in erythrocytes from patients with systemic lupus erythematosus. *J. Exp. Med.*, **155**, 1427–38

122. Minota, S., Terai, C., Nojima, Y., Takano, K., Takai, E., Miyakawa, Y. and Takaku, F. (1984). Low C3b receptor reactivity on erythrocytes from patients with systemic lupus erythematosus detected by immune adherence hemagglutination and radioimmunoassays with monoclonal antibody. *Arthritis Rheum.*, **27**, 1329–35

123. Ross, G. D., Yount, W. J., Walport, M. J., Winfield, J. B., Parker, C. J., Fuller, C. R., Taylor, R. P., Myones, B. L. and Lachmann, P. J. (1985). Disease-associated loss of erythrocyte complement receptors (CR1, C3b receptors) in patients with systemic lupus erythematosus and other diseases involving autoantibodies and/or complement activation. *J. Immunol.*, **135**, 2005–13

123a Walport, M. J., Ng, Y. C., Lachmann, P. J. (1987). Erythrocytes transfused into patients with SLE and haemolytic avaeuia lose complement receptor type 1 from their cell surface. *Clin. Exp. Immunol.*, **59**, 547–54

124. Pangburn, M. K., Schreiber, R. D., Trombold, J. S. and Muller-Eberhard, H. J. (1983). Paroxysmal nocturnal hemoglobinuria: deficiency of factor H-like function of the abnormal erythrocytes. *J. Exp. Med.*, **157**, 1971–80

125. Tausk, F. A., McCutchan, J. A., Spechko, P., Schrieber, R. D. and Gigli, I. (1986). Altered erythrocyte C3b receptor expression, immune complexes, and complement activation in homosexual men in varying risk groups for acquired immune deficiency syndrome. *J. Clin. Invest.*, **78**, 977–82

126. Inada, Y., Kamiyama, M., Kanemitsu, T., Hyman, C. L. and Clark, W. S. (1982). Studies on immune adherence receptor (C3b) receptor activity of human erythrocytes: relation between receptor activity and presence of immune complexes in serum. *Clin. Exp. Immunol.*, **50**, 189–97

127. Marlin, S. D., Morton, C. C., Anderson, D. C. and Springer, T. A. (1986). LFA-1 immunodeficiency disease. Definition of the genetic defect and chromosomal mapping of

A and B subunits of the lymphocyte function-associated antigen (LFA-1) by complementation in hybrid cells. *J. Exp. Med.*, **164**, 855-67

128. Springer, T. A., Telpow, D. B. and Dreyer, W. J. (1985). Sequence homology of the LFA-1 and Mac-1 leukocyte adhesion glycoproteins and unexpected relation to leukocyte interferon. *Nature*, **314**, 540-2

129. Suzuki, S., Argraves, W. S., Pytela, R., Arai, H., Krusius, T., Pierschbacher, M. D. and Ruoslahti, E. (1986). cDNA and amino acid sequences of the cell adhesion protein receptor recognising vitronectin reveal a transmembrane domain and homologies with other adhesion protein receptors. *Proc. Natl. Acad. Sci. USA*, **83**, 8614-18

130. Cosgrove, L. J., Sandrin, M. S., Rajasekariah, P. and McKenzie, I. F. C. (1986). A genomic clone encoding an alpha chain of the OKM 1, LFA-1 and platelet glycoprotein IIb-IIIa molecules. *Proc. Natl. Acad. Sci. USA*, **83**, 752-6

131. Sastre, L., Roman, J. M., Telow, D. B., Dreyer, W. J., Gee, C. E., Larson, R. S., Roberts, T. M. and Springer, T. A. (1986). A partial genomic DNA clone for the subunit of a mouse complement receptor type 3 and cellular adhesion molecule Mac-1. *Proc. Natl. Acad. Sci. USA*, **83**, 5644-8

132. Ross, G. D., Cain, J. A. and Lachmann, P. J. (1985). Membrane complement receptor type three (CR3) has lectin-like properties analogous to bovine conglutinin and functions as a receptor for zymosan and rabbit erythrocytes as well as a receptor for iC3b. *J. Immunol.*, **134**, 3307-15

133. Wright, S. D. and Jong, M. T. C. (1986). Adhesion-promoting receptors on human macrophages recognize *Escherichia coli* by binding to lipopolysaccharide. *J. Exp. Med.*, **164**, 1876-88

134. Lachmann, P. J., Elias, D. E. and Moffett, A. (1972). Conglutinin and immunoconglutinins. In Ingram, D. G. (ed.) *Biological Activities of Complement*. p. 202 (Basel: Karger)

135. Ross, G. D., Thompson, R. A., Walport, M. J., Springer, T. A., Watson, J. V., Ward, R. H. R., Lida, J., Newman, S. L., Harrison, R. A. and Lachmann, P. J. (1985). Characterization of patients with an increased susceptibility to bacterial infections and a genetic deficiency of leukocyte membrane complement antigen LFA-1. *Blood*, **66**, 882-90

136. Micklem, K. J. and Sim, R. B. (1985). Isolation of complement-fragment-iC3b-binding proteins by affinity chromatography. *Biochem. J.*, **231**, 233-6

137. Anderson, D. C., Miller, L. J., Schmalstieg, F. C., Rothlein, R. and Springer, T. A. (1986). Contributions of the Mac-1 glycoprotein family to adherence-dependent granulocyte functions: structure-function assessments employing subunit-specific monoclonal antibodies. *J. Immunol.*, **137**, 15-28

138. Mentzer, S. J., Gromkowski, S. H., Krensky, A. M., Burakoff, S. J. and Martz, E. (1985). LFA-1 membrane molecule in the regulation of homotypic adhesions of human B lymphocytes. *J. Immunol.*, **135**, 9-11

139. Patarroyo, M., Beatty, P. G., Fabre, J. W. and Gahmberg, C. G. (1985). Identification of a cell surface protein complex mediating phorbol ester-induced adhesion (binding) among human mononuclear leukocytes. *Scand. J. Immunol.*, **22**, 171

140. Rothlein, R. and Springer, T. A. (1986). The requirement for lymphocyte function-associated antigen 1 in homotypic leukocyte adhesion stimulated by phorbol ester. *J. Exp. Med.*, **163**, 1132-49

141. Miller, L. J., Schwarting, R. and Springer, T. A. (1986). Regulated expression of the Mac-1, LFA-1, p150,95 glycoprotein family during leukocyte differentiation. *J. Immunol.*, **137**, 2891-900

142. Kay, A. B., Glass, J. and Salter, McG. (1979). Leuco-attractants enhance complement receptors on human phagocytic cells. *Clin. Exp. Immunol.*, **38**, 294-9

143. Fearon, D. T. and Collins, L. A. (1983). Increased expression of C3b receptors on polymorphonuclear leukocytes induced by chemotactic factors and purification procedures. *J. Immunol.*, **130**, 370-5

144. Berger, M., O'Shea, J., Cross, A. S., Folks, T. M., Chused, T. M., Brown, E. J. and Frank, M. M. (1984). Human neutrophils increase expression of C3bi as well as C3b receptors upon activation. *J. Clin. Invest.*, **74**, 1566-77

145. Richerson, H. B., Walsh, G. M., Walport, M. J., Mogbel, R. and Kay, A. B. (1985). Enhancement of human neutrophil complement receptors: a comparison of the rosette

technique with the uptake of radio-labelled anti-CR1 monoclonal antibody. *Clin. Exp. Immunol.*, **62**, 442-8

146. Todd, III R. F., Arnaout A., Rosin, R. E., Crowley, C. A., Peters, W. A. and Babior, B. M. (1984). Subcellular localization of the large subunit of Mol (Mol alpha; formerly gp110) a surface glycoprotein associated with neutrophil adhesion. *J. Clin. Invest.*, **74**, 1280-90

147. Arnaout, M. A., Spits, H., Terhorst, C., Pitt, J. and Todd, III R. F. (1984). Deficiency of a leukocyte surface glycoprotein (LFA-1) on two patients with Mol deficiency. Effects of cell activations on Mol/LFA-1 surface expression in normal and deficient leukocytes. *J. Clin. Invest.*, **74**, 1291-300

148. O'Shea, J.J., Brown, E. J., Seligmann, B. E., Metcalf, J. A., Frank, M. M. and Gallin, J. I. (1985). Evidence for distinct intracellular pools of receptors for C3b and C3bi in human neutrophils. *J. Immunol*, **134**, 2580-7

149. Springer, T. A., Miller, L. J. and Anderson, D. C. (1986). p150, 95 The third member of the MAC-1, LFA-1 human leukocyte adhesion glycoprotein family. *J. Immunol.*, **136**, 240-5

150. Wright, S. D. and Meyer, B. C. (1986). Phorbol esters cause sequential activation and deactivation of complement receptors on polymorphonuclear leukocytes. *J. Immunol.*, **136**, 1759-64

151. Wright, S. D., Detmers, P. A., Jong, M. T. C. and Meyer, B. C. (1986). Interferon-gamma depresses binding of ligand by C3b and C3bi receptors on cultured human monocytes, an effect reversed by fibronectin. *J. Exp. Med.*, **163**, 1245-59

152. Bohnsack, J. F., Kleinman, H. K., Takahashi, T., O'Shea, J. J. and Brown, E. J. (1985). Connective tissue proteins and phagocytic cell function: laminin enhances complement and Fc-mediated phagocytosis by cultured human macrophages. *J. Exp. Med.*, **161**, 912-23

153. Wright, S. D., Craigmyle, L. S. and Silverstein, S. C. (1983). Fibronectin and serum amyloid P component stimulate C3b- and C3bi-mediated phagocytosis in cultured human monocytes. *J. Exp. Med.*, **158**, 1338-43

154. Wright, S. D. and Silverstein, S. C. (1982). Tumor-promoting phorbol esters stimulate C3b and C3b' receptor-mediated phagocytosis in cultured human monocytes. *J. Exp. Med.*, **156**, 1149-64

155. Gallin, J. I. (1985). Leukocyte adherence-related glycoproteins LFA-1, Mol and p150, 95; a new group of monoclonal antibodies, a new disease and a possible opportunity to understand the molecular basis of leukocyte adherence. *J. Infect. Dis.*, **152**, 661-3

156. Hayward, A. R., Leonard, J., Wood, C. B. S., Harvey, B. A. M., Greenwood, M. C. and Soothill, J. F. (1979). Delayed separation of the umbilical cord, widespread infections and defective neutrophil mobility. *Lancet*, **1**, 1099-111

157. Bowen, J., Ochs, H. D. and Wedgwood, R. J. (1979). Chemotaxis and umbilical separation. *Lancet*, **2**, 302

158. Crowley, C. A., Curnutte, J. T., Rosin, R. E., Andrew-Schwartz, J., Gallin, J. I., Klempner, M., Snyderman, R., Southwick, F. S., Stossel, T. P. and Babior, B. M. (1980). An inherited abnormality of neutrophil adhesion: its genetic transmission and its association with a missing protein. *N. Engl. J. Med.*, **302**, 1163-8

159. Abramson, J. S., Mills, E. L., Sawyer, M. K., Regelmann, W. R., Nelson, J. D. and Quie, P. G. (1981). Recurrent infections and delayed separation of the umbilical cord in an infant with abnormal phagocytic cell locomotion and oxidative response during particle phagocytosis. *J. Pediatr.*, **99**, 887-94

160. Bissenden, J. G., Haeney, M. R., Tarlow, M. J. and Thompson, R. A. (1981). Delayed separation of the umbilical cord, severe widespread infections and immunodeficiency. *Arch. Dis. Child.*, **56**, 397-9

161. Buchanan, M. R., Crowley, C. A., Rosin, R. E., Gimbrone, Jnr M. A. and Babior, B. M. (1982). Studies on the interaction between GP-180-deficient neutrophils and vascular endothelium. *Blood*, **60**, 160-5

162. Fischer, A., Trung, P. H., Descamps-Latscha, B., Lisowska Grospierre, B., Gerota, I., Pere, N., Scheinmetzler, C., Durandy, A., Virelixier, J. L. and Griscelli, C. (1983). Bone-marrow transplantation for inborn error of phagocytic cells associated with defective adherence, chemotaxis and oxidative response during opsonized particle phagocytosis. *Lancet*, **2**, 473-6

163. Kobayashi, K. J., Fujita, K., Okino, F. and Kajii, T. (1984). An abnomality of neutrophil

adhesion: autosomal recessive inheritance associated with missing neutrophil glycoproteins. *Pediatrics*, **73**, 606-10

164. Davies, E. G., Isaacs, D. and Levinsky, R. J. (1982). Defective immune interferon production and natural killer activity associated with poor neutrophil mobility and delayed umbilical cord separation. *Clin. Exp. Immunol.*, **50**, 454-60

165. Bowen, T. J., Ochs, H. D., Altman, L. C., Price, T. H., Van Epps, D. P., Brautigan, D. L., Rosin, R. E., Perkins, W. D., Babior, B. N. M., Klebanoff, S. J. and Wedgwood, R. J. (1982). Severe recurrent bacterial infections associated with defective adherence and chemotaxis in two patients with neutrophils deficient in a cell-associated glycoprotein. *J. Pediatr.*, **101**, 932-9

166. Beatty, P. G., Ochs, H. D., Harlan, J. M., Price, T. H., Rosen, H., Taylor, R. F., Hansen, J. A. and Klebanoff, S. J. (1984). Absence of monoclonal antibody-defined protein complex in a boy with abnormal leukocyte function. *Lancet*, **1**, 535-7

167. Arnaout, M. A., Pitt, J., Cohen, H. J., Melamed, J., Rosen, F. S. and Colten, H. R. (1982). Deficiency of a granulocyte-membrane glycoprotein (gp150) in a boy with recurrent bacterial infections. *N. Engl. J. Med.*, **306**, 696-9

168. Anderson, D. C., Schmalsteig, F. C., Finegold, M. H. J., Hughes, B. J., Rothlein, R., Miller, L. J., Kohl, S., Tosi, M. F., Jacobs, R. L., Waldrop, T. C., Goldman, A. S., Shearer, W. T. and Springer, T. A. (1985). The severe and moderate phenotypes of hereditary Mac-1 LFA-1 deficiency: their quantitative definition and relation to leukocyte dysfunction and clinical features. *J. Infect. Dis.*, **152**, 668-89

169. Anderson, D. C., Schmalsteig, F. C., Kohl, S., Arnaout, M. A., Tosi, M. F., Dana, N., Buffone, G. J., Hughes, B. J., Brinkley, B. R., Dickey, W. D., Abramson, J. S., Springer, T., Boxer, L. A., Hollers, J. M. and Smith, C. W. (1984). Abnormalities of polymorphonuclear leukocyte function associated with a heritable deficiency of high molecular weight surface glycoproteins (GP138): common relationship to diminished cell adherence. *J. Clin. Invest.*, **74**, 536-51

170. Thompson, R. A., Candy, D. C. A. and McNeish, A. I. (1984). Familial defect of polymorph neutrophil phagocytosis associated with absence of a surface glycoprotein antigen (OKM1). *Clin. Exp. Immunol.*, **58**, 229-36

171. Dana, N., Todd, R. F. III, Pitt, J., Springer, T. A. and Arnaout, M. A. (1984). Deficiency of a surface membrane glycoprotein (Mol) in man. *J. Clin. Invest.*, **73**, 153-9

172. Sanchez-Madrid, F., Nagy, J. A., Robbins, E., Simon, P. and Springer, T. A. (1983). A human leukocyte differentiation antigen family with distinct alpha subunits and a common beta subunit: the lymphocyte-function associated antigen (LFA-1), the C3bi complement receptor (OKM1/Mac-1) and the p150,95 molecule. *J. Exp. Med.*, **158**, 1785-98

173. Springer, T. A., Thompson, W. S., Miller, L. J., Schmalsteig, F. C. and Anderson, D. C. (1984). Inherited deficiency of the Mac-1, LFA-1, p 150,95 glycoprotein family and its molecular basis. *J. Exp. Med.*, **160**, 1901-18

174. Fischer, A., Durandy, A., Sterkers, G. and Griscelli, C. (1986). Role of the LFA-1 molecule in cellular interactions required for antibody production in humans. *J. Immunol.*, **136**, 3198-202

175. Kohl, S., Springer, T. A., Schmalsteig, F. C., Loo, L. S. and Anderson, D. C. (1984). Defective natural killer cytotoxicity and polymorphonuclear leukocyte antibody-dependent cellular cytotoxicity in patients with LFA-1/OKM-1 deficiency. *J. Immunol.*, **133**, 2972-8

176. Harlan, J. M., Killen P. D., Senecal, F. M., Schwartz, B. R., Yee, E. K., Taylor, R. F., Beatty, P. G., Price, T. H. and Ochs, H. D. (1985). The role of neutrophil membrane glycoprotein GP-150 in neutrophil adherence to endothelium *in vitro*. *Blood*, **66**, 167-78

177. Ross, G. D., Newman, S. L., Lambris, J. D., Devery-Pocius, J., Cain, J. A. and Lachmann, P. J. (1983). Generation of three different fragments of bound C3 with purified factor I or serum. II. Location of binding sites in the C3 fragments for factors B and H, complement receptors, and bovine conglutinin. *J. Exp. Med.*, **158**, 334-52

Index